The Healthy Mind Cookbook

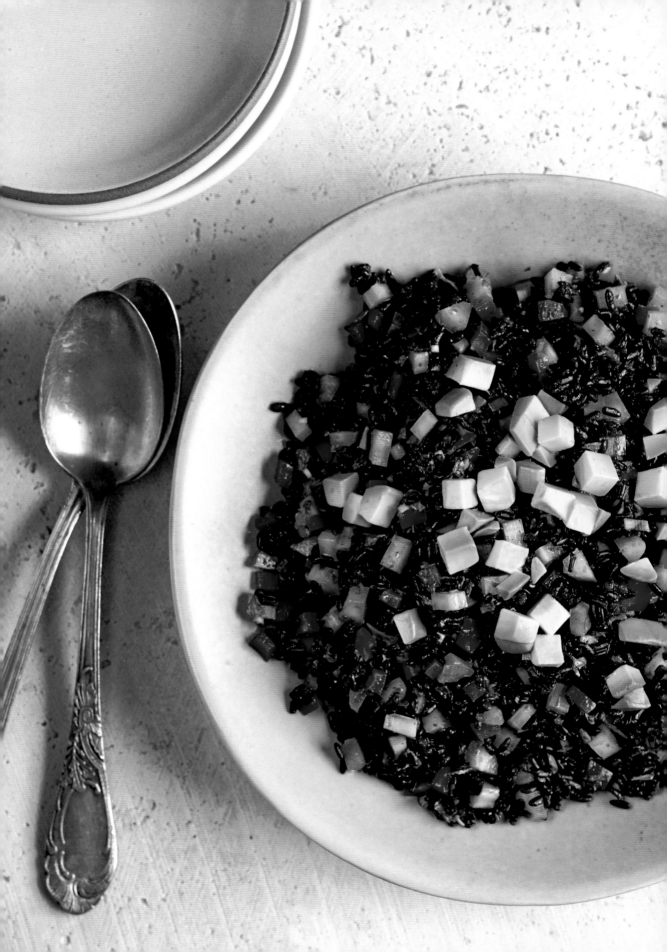

THE
Healthy Mind
COOKBOOK

Big-Flavor Recipes to Enhance Brain Function,
Mood, Memory, and Mental Clarity

Rebecca Katz WITH Mat Edelson

PHOTOGRAPHY BY MAREN CARUSO

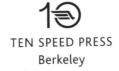

TEN SPEED PRESS
Berkeley

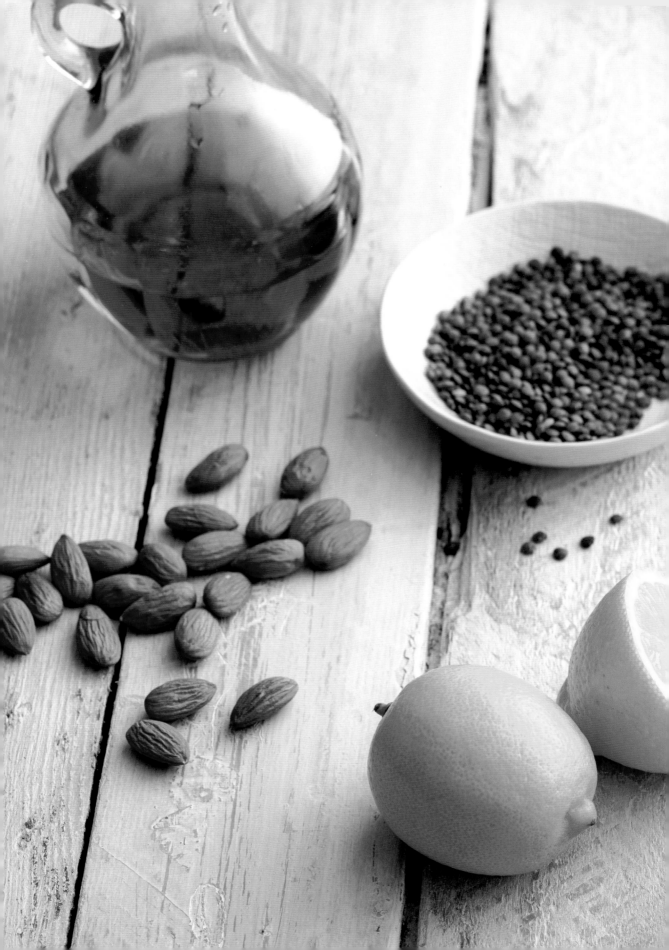

Contents

CHAPTER 8

Dollops 163

CHAPTER 9

Tonics and Elixirs 187

CHAPTER 10

Sweet Bites 209

Acknowledgments

A COMMUNITY OF BIG THINKERS and doers gave fully of their time and talents to make this book all that it could be. Together we'd like to thank:

Jeremy Katz, our wonderful agent, friend, and advocate who supports us with sage advice and humor, and Simon Katz, for contributing another inspiring culinary concoction to this collection.

Julie and Stan Burford, and of course, Josie, the wonder dog. A huge culinary hug to all of you for buoying up Mat and myself with many bright ideas, nourishing meals, wisdom, and a major dollop of moral support.

The talented people at Ten Speed Press: We thank publisher Aaron Wehner, and editorial director Julie Bennett, for their dedication to this project; Melissa Moore, editor extraordinaire; Kelly Snowden, the editor who brought this book to the finish line with style and finesse; Chloe Rawlins, for going the extra mile to deliver yet another masterful and beautiful design; Emma Campion, Betsy Stromberg, and Toni Tajima, for lending their keen creative eye during the photo shoots; Clancy Drake, for her extraordinary copyediting; Jean Blomquist, our proof reader, for crossing the t's and dotting the i's; Hannah Rahill, Michele Crim, and Ashley Matuzak, for their sales and marketing expertise; and Lorraine Woodcheke, for her public relations wizardry.

For the beautiful photography, we thank photographer Maren Caruso and her fantastic team, including food stylists Christine Wolheim and Kim Kissling, and prop stylist Kerrie Sherrel Walsh, who created the lovely images that grace the pages of this book.

REBECCA THANKS . . . Catherine McConkie, whose graciousness, creativity, culinary talent, and amazing taste buds inform every recipe in this book. Jen Yasis, whose diligence, hard work, infectious laugh, and positive attitude were essential ingredients in all aspects of this manuscript; Heidi Snyder, CHN, MS, NC, for her expert nutritional analysis that accompanies each recipe; and Anteo Quiroz, for tracking all the copious amounts of research involved in the making of this book.

A huge thank you to my co-author Mat Edelson. This is our fourth book together, and this time around you've amazed me by delving into the science of the brain while recovering from a broken back. You're a brilliant writer no matter what the circumstances.

Thank you to my friend and colleague Andrew Weil, MD, for reinforcing that cooking and sharing food should be fun and enjoyed.

Thank you to my Commonweal family, where the Healing Kitchens Institute (HKI) calls home. Michael Lerner, for continued support, guidance, and belief in my work; Waz Thomas, Claire Heart, Sadja Greenwood, MD, Oren Slozberg, Arlene Allsman, Kate Holcombe, Jenepher Stowell, Mimi Mindel, Shelia Oppenheimer, and the rest of the Commonweal community, for making Commonweal such a special and magical place for people to find healing and nourishment.

Thank you to Jim Gordon, MD, founder and director of the Center for Mind Body Medicine, and the staff and faculty of Food as Medicine. A special thank you to Kathie Madonna Swift, MS, RD, LDN, goddess of nutrition, for all that you've taught me over the years with grace and kindness.

Jo Cooper, dear friend, colleague, and my marketing impresario. You are a treasure! Tara Blazona and Olga Katzneslson of Postcard Communications for your help in getting the word out.

Thank you to the cheerleaders, friends, and colleagues including Stefanie Sacks, MS, for your friendship and inviting me to play culinary ping-pong on your radio show *Stirring the Pot*, Marti Wolfson; Jo Cessna; Caroline Nation; Jeanne Wallace, PhD; Fredi Kronenberg, PhD; Donald Abrams, MD; Sandy and Harlan Kleiman; Dale E. Bredesen, MD; Toni Brooks, MFT; Eric Gower; Kathryn Graham Wilson; Joyce Aronowitz; Jennifer Omholt; Paul and Vicki Remer; Wendy Remer; and Jill Leiner.

Super special thanks and a huge hug to my Ma, Barbara Katz; my brother, Jeff; Harry and Amelia; Andy and Asako; and my grandchildren Brandon and Chloe Hannah, for all that you have taught me about living in the moment. No doubt, the recipes in this book would never have been completed without the help of my kitchen dogs, Bella and Lola. Of course my husband, Gregg Kellogg, for his unwavering support for my work; and to my father, the late Jay Katz, who continues to inspire me, and whose love of food seasons each page of this book.

MAT THANKS . . . Normally, book acknowledgments are all about the people who helped put a book together. We'll get to them in a moment. First, a nod to all those folks who put me back together after Humpty-Dumpty fell (jumped) off the high-diving board and managed to break his back (and, yes, there was water in the pool). Without them, there is no book. To the ER/neurology docs at Largo (FL) Medical, you saved my legs; every step I take, I have you to thank. Ditto the neurology team at Johns Hopkins. And I had the Florence Nightingale of nurses in my partner and love in all things fine and dandy, Deb; it's amazing how far a little Gold Bond powder can go when you're stuck in a body brace in the middle of summer.

Now for the book. Duffy, your work with the Culinary Pharmacy was a game changer. Thanks for stepping up in a pinch. Rebecca, this is our fourth go-round at the rodeo, and it only gets better. Your way with food and people is unparalleled, and you are changing the world for the better. As for the numerous physicians, researchers, and wellness pros out there who freely gave of their time, knowledge, and wisdom, you have my heartfelt appreciation.

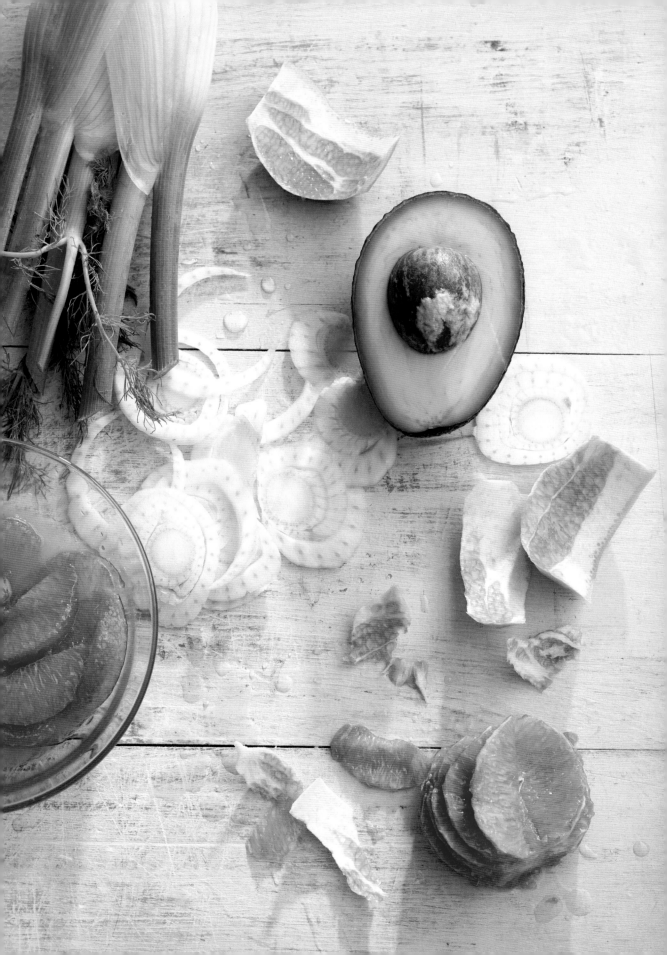

Introduction

SOMETIMES, WRITING A BOOK IS CATHARTIC. My father, Jay, died of dementia in his eighties, after struggling with the disease for a decade. Ever since, I felt like I was on a timetable, that my mind had an expiration date of age seventy or so. It wasn't a pleasant way to feel, but justified, I thought, given my paternal genetics.

And then I began researching for this book on the connections between brain health and food—an effort that would have yielded far different results if I had embarked on this adventure even five years earlier. For in the last few years, the science regarding food and its impact on mind, mood, and, yes, memory, has exploded. Put simply, what we put on the end of our fork definitely affects the brain in a myriad of ways. For me, this notion is incredibly liberating. Is it a cure-all? Maybe yes, maybe no: time, as they say, will tell. But I'm an optimist by nature, and I believe the science suggests that food may well be nature's answer to the host of brain maladies that affects so many of us.

I'm talking things such as depression, ADHD, forgetfulness, agitation, brain fog, fatigue . . . the things we deal with every day that may be the biting flies on our otherwise pristine beach. These ailments nag away at us to the point that many of us consider them an inevitable part of life.

But they don't have to be. I'm not here to knock conventional medicine—it certainly can be crucial in addressing mental health issues—but my kind of medicine—food— absolutely has its place at the table.

Let's consider for a moment the tech-revved world many of us (and certainly our kids) live in. At work, our gadgets keep us constantly on call; daily we spend much of our mental energies stemming the tide. Our youth are plugged in, too, video-stimulated to the max, their brains afire with input. Either way, there's no downtime: little opportunity for the mind to relax, rest, and recover (and that's not even including the lack of sleep endemic to the population).

So we're asking more and more of our brain: we're demanding it be smart, alert, adept, adaptive . . . in short, to be with the program at all times.

That's a tall order for any organ, let alone one that often isn't getting the right fuel for the job. If the brain is our premier organ, there's little doubt it needs premium fuel, the ol' 93 at the pump. But a lot of folks who own premium cars are tempted to stick in lower grade fuel and save a half-buck a gallon, because after all, gas is gas, right?

Not exactly. Keep putting in 87 instead of 93, and pretty soon the engine knocks, the timing goes off, and instead of being able to quickly accelerate to information superhighway speed, you're left in the slow lane wondering where you put your glasses when all the while they're on top of your head.

This book is all about giving your brain the right fuel to do the job you want it to do. Now here's the fun part: You can do it with walnuts. You can do it with blueberries. You can do it with wild salmon. You can do it with kale. You can do it eighty-five different ways (actually far more; eighty-five refers to the number of ingredients in this book, but the number of combinations is exponential). We're talking ingredients with oodles of taste and flavor in addition to the nutrients the brain craves.

I've come to see this book as a way to help you make friends with your brain, turning it into a trusted ally instead of a capricious companion. The inability to remember Aunt Sally's husband's name at a wedding, or to recall the year the first moonshot landed—for many of us, daily battles with our brains are a given.

But what if I told you that you could eat certain foods to help you ace the exam, or be at your sharpest for a big meeting, or be relaxed at that first confab with the in-laws? It's not science fiction, but science fact. Add in some culinary wisdom and what you've got are fantastic foods that are as delicious as they are brain boosting.

Talk about empowering! For the first time in the long history of gastronomy, science has gotten behind the plate to confirm and expand upon what many have long thought: that mint can refresh, ginger can invigorate, cinnamon can improve memory, basil can improve mental clarity, and much more. How much more? Go to the Culinary Pharmacy on page 9 and you'll find peer-reviewed scientific studies backing the claims for every ingredient in the book.

Now I know there's a temptation, at least when it comes to the brain, to put off paying attention to its needs. That dovetails with the commonly held belief that brain problems, notably regarding memory, don't start until we're elderly.

This is not the case. Research has shown that the roots of many memory problems begin in our twenties and thirties, which is my way of saying it's never too early to pay attention to how we're nourishing our brains. For me, the notion that what I eat can positively impact my mind is incredibly freeing. I no longer feel that I'm a prisoner to my genetics. Instead, I have a measure of control over both my future and my present brain health.

The same holds true for you. Few things can have greater importance in (or impact on) your life than the decision to properly nourish your and your family's brain health. The joy is in discovering that great nutrition and great taste can coexist delightfully on the plate. How do we get there? Well, the best way is to think of you and me as a team; together we're going to take an exciting journey across the threshold of the kitchen to the place where all this culinary magic takes place, right at the stove.

Because in your mind, that's the place you want to be. Now, let's make it happen.

CHAPTER 1

Your Brain on Food

WHEN I THINK OF THE BRAIN—my brain, *anybody's* brain—I'm both dumbfounded and astounded: Dumbfounded because essentially a lump (three pounds) of mostly (60 percent) fat can be the seat of our emotions, our heartbeat, our memories, our respiration, our learning, our consciousness, and, perhaps, our soul. Astounded because among that fat lie some 100 billion brain cells (neurons). If you want to wrap your head around that number, think, as neuroscientist Frank Amthor notes, of all the stars in our galaxy—including the ones you can't see with the naked eye—and you're getting close. Kind of. Maybe. If that isn't enough, each neuron talks to others using numerous branches called dendrites and axons; if you want an image, recall those old-time movies where there was a switchboard operator plugging line "A" into "your party"—line "B"—and, well, there's a stick figure drawing of your brain in action.

That the brain and its function has long been a mystery is no mystery. From the Bible through the Renaissance, from Socrates to Shakespeare to today, our great minds found their understanding of the brain's properties to be as ethereal as gossamer wings. "Everything we do, every thought we've ever had, is produced by the human brain," says astrophysicist Neil deGrasse Tyson. "But exactly how it operates remains one of the biggest unsolved mysteries, and it seems the more we probe its secrets, the more surprises we find."

Many of those surprises come in the scientific connections between food and the various workings of the brain. Type "food and brain" into the National Library of Medicine's encyclopedic database and you come up with roughly 32,000 peer-reviewed studies—and the curve is clearly accelerating as nearly half of those studies have occurred in the past ten years. Food and mood, food and memory, food and learning—all are being investigated, and there's a growing body of evidence suggesting that what we eat either primarily affects our brain or has secondary effects (for example, whatever you eat that's heart healthy also may lower the risk of stroke, which is definitely a brain condition).

Here we take a look at some of those food-brain connections.

Stress, Anxiety, Depression, and Food

Let's face it: most of us don't treat our brains with kid gloves. Between blowing off sleep, multitasking to the max, and eating poorly, we put our brains under a tremendous amount of stress. Now, our brains are equipped to handle stress through a mechanism called the fight-or-flight response. When the stress happens suddenly (like when you're driving along and you slam on the brakes to avoid an accident), what you notice, after you've done a body check, is that your heart is pounding, your mouth is dry, and you've broken out into a sweat. That's the result of the hypothalamus—an area deep in your primitive brain—sending out a signal to the adrenal glands to essentially "pump up the volume" and shoot a hormone called cortisol, and a few neurotransmitters like norepinephrine and dopamine into your system.

Cortisol et al. are what allowed your ancestors to outrun a saber-toothed tiger (for at least a few seconds, until they reached safety), and, in the modern world, make for those occasional sensational headlines like "Wife Lifts Car Off Husband." But the fight-or-flight response—and our adrenal system—was never intended to be on full time. That way lies burnout and more. Researchers at Emory University noted that depressed people often had extremely high levels of cortisol in their blood. Another study from Canadian researchers published in *Brain and Cognition* showed that stress hormones negatively impacted cognition, our ability to process and remember information. If stress continues long enough, it can, as the Latin root of the word *distress* suggests, "pull us apart," destroying brain cells in the hippocampus, the memory-creating center of the brain.

Fortunately, to a great degree we can combat stress. Exercise and mind-body work such as yoga and/or meditation certainly help. And food can be a great boon to relaxation. Now here's where you need to follow the bouncing ball. When cortisol floods the body constantly, it causes the body to break down the amino acid tryptophan more rapidly. This is decidedly *not* a good thing for your mood, because the higher the levels of tryptophan that stay in the body, the more tryptophan there is to convert into—wait for it—serotonin. Serotonin is the brain's happy hormone. So, under certain conditions, more tryptophan = more serotonin = better mood. I say "certain conditions" because just eating a ton of turkey (like at Thanksgiving dinner) won't do the trick, because tryptophan is just one of many amino acids vying for the brain's attention and absorption. What you're looking for is foods that have a high ratio of tryptophan in their overall amino acid profile, which increases the odds that tryptophan will make it through the so-called blood/brain barrier and be usable by the brain. You'll find that in, of all places, pumpkin and sesame seeds (which, not coincidentally, are in this book). Another way of keeping tryptophan in the system is by making sure you get a larger proportion of vegetables on your plate with each protein-filled meal. According to nutrition expert Dr. Michael Greger, the carbs in plant foods are known to cause an insulin release that, Greger writes, "causes our muscles to take up many of the non-tryptophan amino acids as fuel, potentially leaving our tryptophan first in line for brain access."

Another mood enhancer may be omega-3 fatty acids. These are found in cold-water fish, such as wild salmon, and in walnuts. Researchers looking at Japanese culture noted a marked lack of depression (as much as 90 percent less than among Americans); they also discovered that the Japanese, on average, ate fifteen times more omega-3s than Americans. Investigators in a large study in Montreal found that supplementing the diet with omega-3s brought relief to some patients with major depression who did not have anxiety issues. Other investigators, including Dr. Andrew Weil, cite a diet rich in anti-inflammatory ingredients, such as sardines and extra-virgin olive oil, to be helpful in reducing depression, and Ohio State researchers found that fighting inflammation with omega-3s lowered anxiety in some students.

Memory, Cognition, Learning, and Food

If there's ever been an elephant lurking under the living room rug, it's the topic of memory, especially faulty memory. It wasn't long ago that experiencing a fading memory as one aged was considered inevitable. But that notion is undergoing a critical review, driven by a concept called neural regeneration (aka neurogenesis). Scientists for decades believed that the adult brain was incapable of adding new brain cells, or neurons, to replace those that were damaged or had died off. Recent discoveries have many of them now thinking the opposite: that new cells can be produced, notably in parts of the brain, such as the hippocampus, connected with learning. (Interestingly from a food viewpoint, the other area of the brain that appears to generate new neurons throughout life is in the olfactory bulb, which is where our sense of smell resides.)

Can we supercharge this regeneration process through food, and preserve our minds? Research is suggesting it's possible. For example, consuming omega-3s is linked to greater activity of a chemical known as brain-derived neurotropic factor (BDNF). BDNF is believed to be responsible for kick-starting the growth of new neurons. A Spanish study found that, in addition to omega-3s, foods rich in vitamin E and flavanols (such as nuts and seeds, broccoli, and citrus fruits) increased BDNF levels, as did following a Mediterranean diet rich in walnuts and almonds. As to where you should get your vitamin E—pills versus food—Dr. Neal Barnard is adamant you go with the latter. "Vitamin E is protective," he says, "but in a pill it's only generally one form, alpha-tocopherol; but if you eat walnuts, you get all seven forms."

Diet may also help counteract naturally occurring molecules within the body that attack memory and cognition. One such molecule is homocysteine, which is a by-product of the protein-building process. A study of 1,140 people aged fifty to seventy in Baltimore found that higher homocysteine levels were "associated with worse function across a broad range of cognitive domains." The antidote may be increasing your intake of vitamins B6, B9 (folate), and B12. Oxford researchers found that when they gave this vitamin regimen to people with mild cognitive impairment, their homocysteine levels dropped greatly and, over a two-year period, their cognitive testing scores jumped by up to 70 percent.

And again, don't forget exercise. University of Pittsburgh neuroscience researcher Kirk Erickson notes that "exercise activates neurotransmitters and growth factors that affect new neurons in the brain. Exercise can influence gene expression." He adds, "Throughout our lifespan our brain remains plastic, modifiable, and the things we do in our life, exercise and what we eat, affect the health and plasticity of the brain."

The Mighty Methylators and Detoxification

The B vitamins, notably B6, B9, and B12, also play a huge role in the process known as methylation, which controls the expression and repair of our DNA. Deficiencies in these B vitamins can lead to breakdowns in methylation and thence to improper DNA expression and repair, which in turn may help cause a whole host of mental issues including "depression, pediatric cognitive dysfunction, dementia, and stroke," says Dr. Mark Hyman. He adds that methylation is "the key to detoxification," because the process keeps a major player in detoxification, the super antioxidant glutathione, circulating in the body. Hyman also notes that methylation reduces inflammation and keeps neurotransmitters balanced. His suggestion to keep methylation functioning well is to consume plenty of dark, leafy greens, including kale, Swiss chard, spinach, and collards.

And Now a Word from Our Second Brain . . .

And you thought you only had *one* brain? Au contraire. Columbia University professor Michael Gershon came up with the term "the second brain" to describe the actions of the gut and enteric nervous system (ENS). The description is apt, for just as the brain in our head has neurotransmitters and nerve cells, so too does the gut—in the enteric nervous system. (The word *enteric* means "of or having to do with the intestines.")

The fascinating thing about the ENS is that though it works to control much of the digestion in your gut, it definitely is impacted by what's going on in the brain inside your head. The two are connected by the vagus nerve, which winds from the brain stem through to the abdomen. The vagus nerve controls our parasympathetic nervous system (PNS), which rides herd, along with the ENS, on digestion. There's another nervous system, the sympathetic nervous system (SNS), which controls the aforementioned fight-or-flight response. The important thing to remember—at least when it comes to digestion—is that when fight-or-flight is engaged, it shuts down digestion (which makes sense: if you're running for your life, you don't have time to chow down, or energy for any metabolic function that's not going to save your life this very minute).

Under normal, relaxed conditions, just *thinking* about food is enough to get our digestion rolling, as anyone who has ever opened a menu, read a few words, and found their mouth watering can attest. This so-called "cephalic" stage of eating is amazing.

"You may secrete as much as 40 percent of the hydrochloric acid and digestive enzymes needed to break down the foods you eat *before* you consume a single ounce of food," write Dr. Gerard Mullin and Kathie Madonna Swift.

But when we're stressed, and the sympathetic nervous system has the upper hand, signals to the vagus nerve get disrupted, and digestion all down the line suffers. When stress is chronic, a dangerous cycle begins as we try to take in the nutrients we need for a healthy body and brain (that's why you're reading this book, yes?), yet stress impairs our GI tract and keeps it from assimilating those very nutrients. Acid reflux, irritable bowel disease—these may well be the result if you're not treating your second brain very well. As a consequence, your first and principal brain suffers. So do both your brains a favor: before you eat, take a moment, and a few deep breaths. Then let the eating—and healing—begin!

Brain Science and Mindful Choices

It's easy to get overwhelmed by the sheer volume of science surrounding the brain and food. Even I get dazed trying to wrap my head around all the studies and new information that seem to be coming out on an almost daily basis. My advice? Take the science with a bit of a "gee-whiz!" approach as opposed to thinking, "I have to understand this *all,* right now!"

I experience the science as both engaging and motivating: I'm excited that so many researchers are interested in this field, and I'm thrilled that food and cooking may really make a difference in how our minds function. Now it becomes a matter of getting behind the stove and doing it, and I'll be with you all the way.

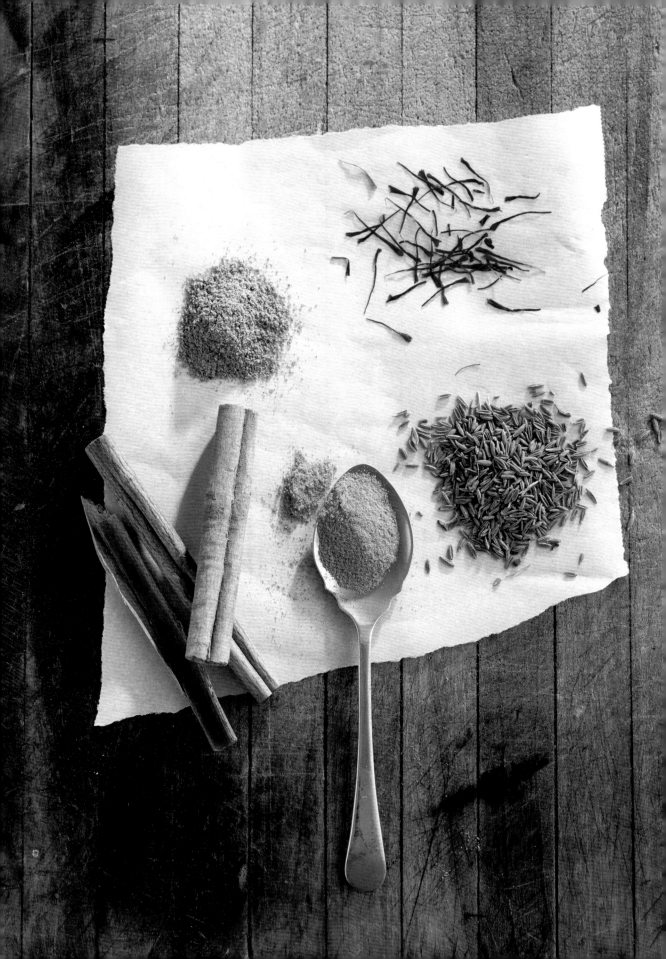

CHAPTER 2

The Culinary Pharmacy

THE CULINARY PHARMACY, open 24/7, is the place where you can dive in headfirst to the latest science behind nearly every ingredient in the book. The information here has been drawn from hundreds of peer-reviewed studies conducted with humans, animals, and in the lab, looking at the connection between foods and the brain. Though the pace of this research is increasing, and more suggestive links are occurring all the time, the science hasn't yet reached the place where many definitive conclusions can be drawn between diet and brain health. Still, it is worthwhile—and fascinating—to see what science has uncovered to date—always remembering the picture is an evolving one.

It's a delight to find out that foods you always thought were delicious also turn out to be power-packed with brain-healthy nutrients. And there are surprises as well: betcha didn't know that tiny little pepitas—aka pumpkin seeds—have a triple kick of potassium, magnesium, and calcium, which have all been associated with delaying cognitive decline and boosting mood.

Everything from allspice to yogurt is included here—some eighty-plus ingredients in all—with notes on the roles they play in helping memory, mood, sleep, energy, and more. This is one of those sections of the book you'll find yourself sampling time and again. It's almost as addictive as the food itself. Enjoy.

ALLSPICE. *Cognitive functioning. Memory. Mental energy.* This fragrant spice, which comes from the dried fruit of the pimenta tree of Central America, serves up a bevy of important vitamins and minerals. It's rich in vitamin C and vitamin B9 (folate), both of which may improve brain functioning as we get older. Riboflavin is here, too, and that's been shown to help reduce fatigue. Allspice also has magnesium, a mineral that is an important part of diets that can help prevent cognitive decline.

ALMONDS. *Cognitive functioning. Mood. Vascular functioning.* Almonds may help your body fight inflammation in ways that can boost mood and slow the mental decline that comes with age. They also may raise levels of the neurotransmitter serotonin, associated with fewer down moods and less depression. Plus, almonds are a heart-healthy food, and that's a boon for the brain, too. People with risk factors for cardiovascular disease show poorer brain functioning than those at lower risk—and the differences start to emerge as young as age thirty-five.

ANCHOVIES. *Cognitive functioning. Focus. Memory. Mental energy. Mood.* These fish are a great source of brain-boosting vitamins and minerals. Vitamin B12 is essential for basic cognitive functioning; deficiencies can hurt concentration, memory, and mood. The mineral calcium can help slow the onset of brain diseases. Plus, anchovies are rich in omega-3 fatty acids, which can boost the performance of brain neurons.

ASPARAGUS. *Cognitive functioning. Mental energy. Mood.* When stored and prepared correctly, asparagus spears can be a rich source of brain-boosting nutrients. They are loaded with vitamin B1 (thiamin), which boosts mood and energy levels, and vitamin B2 (riboflavin), which reduces fatigue. Asparagus also boasts antioxidant and anti-inflammatory nutrients that may help slow cognitive decline. And it's a heart-healthy vegetable, and improved cardiovascular health also facilitates brain functioning.

AVOCADO. *Cognitive functioning. Mood.* When folks hear about carotenoids, they usually think of reddish vegetables such as carrots. But avocados are full of them, too, and carotenoids may improve brain performance and prevent cognitive decline, with a stronger association suggesting it keeps depression at bay. The avocado also has lots of the healthiest fats out there—the kind that can keep inflammation under control and lower the risk of heart disease. Those heart-healthy benefits are linked with better brain performance as well.

BASIL. *Cognitive functioning. Healthy sleep. Memory. Mental energy.* Basil boasts a pair of brain-friendly ingredients, as it's rich in flavonoids and magnesium. Flavonoids have been linked to memory gains and higher scores on cognitive tests. In animals, higher magnesium levels in the brain have been shown to improve memory and learning skills, while in humans the mineral promotes more of the deep sleep that helps increase energy levels.

BEEF AND BISON (GRASS-FED). *Cognitive functioning. Focus. Memory. Mental energy.* Grass-fed beef and bison are the healthy choice here, as they contain more of the vitamins and omega-3 fatty acids that can boost our brain's performance. The red meats are rich in a pair of memory-boosting nutrients—vitamin B12 and zinc. They're also high in vitamin B6, which boosts our mental focus and attention, and vitamin B3, which has been linked to more mental energy. Bison, especially, is an important source of iron, and iron deficiencies are associated with a number of cognitive problems.

BEETS. *Blood flow. Cognitive functioning. Mood.* Beets are a brain food of the first order. They're high in nitrites, which have been shown to increase blood flow in parts of the brain related to executive functioning. They've got lots of folate, or vitamin B9, which may aid cognitive functioning and delay a descent into dementia as we age. Beets are also rich in carotenoids, especially the ones called betalains. These may help boost brain functioning and stave off depression.

BELL PEPPERS. *Cognitive functioning. Mood.* These colorful members of the nightshade family are loaded with powerful carotenoids, which are linked with improved brain function and reduced depression. They're also a great source of vitamin B9 (folate), another performance booster for the brain. Additionally, bell peppers deliver a good chunk of vitamin C, which may elevate our mood and help us stay sharp as we get older.

BISON (*see* Beef and Bison)

BLACK COD. *Cognitive functioning.* Found in the northern Pacific, this deepwater fish (which, technically, isn't a member of the cod family) is also known as sablefish. It's a rich source of omega-3 fatty acids, which may reduce the risk of cognitive impairment as we get older and may even help improve brain functioning. Plus, black cod has lots of vitamin D, which is strongly linked to slowing cognitive decline.

BLUEBERRIES. *Cognitive functioning. Memory. Neuronal health.* Blueberries are a boon for the brain. The flavonoids they deliver help delay cognitive decline in older people. Blueberry consumption may also improve memory and help neurons survive. This latter result seems to be related to the high level of antioxidants in blueberries, which helps promote a balanced metabolism that enhances nerve communication.

BROCCOLI. *Cognitive functioning. Memory.* Broccoli is one of the top sources out there for vitamin K, which appears to boost verbal recall. The B vitamins are here in abundance as well, especially folate, which is linked with better mental functioning and, as we get older, the prevention of dementia. Broccoli is also great for cardiovascular health, and that in turn promotes healthy brain functioning.

CABBAGE. *Cognitive functioning. Memory.* The cruciferous vegetables are among the healthiest of food options, and cabbages are no exception. One recent study of fruits and vegetables singles out cabbages (along with nuts and root vegetables) as especially powerful brain foods. Cabbage has lots of vitamin K, which has been shown to boost certain aspects of memory. Red cabbages, especially, have antioxidant phytochemicals that protect neurons from damage caused by oxidative stress.

CARDAMOM. *Focus. Mental energy.* This rich tropical spice offers generous amounts of a number of key nutrients and minerals. The mineral trio of potassium, calcium, and magnesium may prevent cognitive decline later in life. Cardamom boasts the B vitamins as well, most notably riboflavin, which can reduce fatigue, and thiamin, which can boost energy and concentration. Interestingly, cardamom is a key ingredient in a traditional herbal remedy used in India, and a recent study showed that this remedy might have promise for preventing cognitive decline.

CARROTS. *Cognitive functioning. Learning. Memory.* Carrots aren't just about your eyesight. Recent studies on vitamin A—carrots are chock-full of the stuff—show that it may boost learning skills and may help us maintain our thinking skills as we age. This latter finding is echoed in a study that found better brain functioning in people who ate more root vegetables. Carrots are also rich in vitamin K, a memory enhancer. They are also one of the most heart-healthy vegetables, and a healthy cardiovascular system promotes better cognition.

CASHEWS. *Healthy sleep. Learning. Memory. Mental energy. Mood.* Cashews are a great source of two brain-boosting minerals, zinc and magnesium. Zinc is important because low levels of the mineral are associated with depression, and it may improve memory as well, while magnesium has been shown to help better regulate sleeping patterns and may improve learning skills. Cashews also contain the B vitamin thiamin, which, in women, has been linked with more mental energy and better moods. Plus, the vitamin E here is vital, as low levels of the vitamin are linked with poorer cognition.

CAULIFLOWER. *Cognitive functioning. Memory. Mood.* The health value of cruciferous vegetables such as cauliflower is a big topic in science these days, and it's no wonder. Cauliflower is a great source of the antioxidant vitamin C, which is good not only for the overall health of your brain, but possibly also for your spirits—it may elevate your mood. The vitamin K in cauliflower may keep your mind sharp in your older years; it may also help boost your memory. There's also quite a bit of folate in cauliflower, and that B vitamin boosts overall cognitive functioning.

CHERRIES. *Cognitive functioning. Healthy sleep.* Cherries are a rare natural source of the hormone melatonin, which helps regulate our sleep. Indeed, researchers have found that cherry consumption can help increase both the length and quality of our rest. It may also tame insomnia. Cherries are also an antioxidant powerhouse, delivering the vitamin C we need to keep our brains functioning at their best.

CHICKEN (ORGANIC OR PASTURE-RAISED). *Cognitive functioning. Memory.* A team of Italian scientists recently measured the health-promoting ingredients in three different types of chicken—the traditional grocery store variety, the ones labeled organic, and "organic-plus" ones that were genuinely pasture-raised. The latter two had higher levels of the omega-3 fatty acids, while the pasture-raised variety also was higher in healthy antioxidants. Both ingredients may well help brain functioning. In addition, organic chicken is a good source of the B vitamins that may help to boost your memory and improve your mental focus.

CHICKPEAS. *Cognitive functioning. Healthy sleep. Learning. Memory.* Chickpeas deliver their antioxidant benefits through an array of phytonutrients and flavonoids that may also help boost our memories and enhance brain functioning. Also known as garbanzo beans, chickpeas are a great source of folate and magnesium. Folate has been shown to boost scores on cognitive tests, while magnesium has been shown to boost learning skills in animals and improve sleep quality in humans.

CHILE PEPPERS. *Cognitive functioning. Learning.* Capsaicin is the compound that gives chile peppers their heat. It may also fire up your brain, judging by studies in animals showing a capsaicin-fueled boost in cognitive functioning. Chile peppers are also a great source of vitamin A, which can boost learning skills and may help stave off mental decline over the long haul.

CHOCOLATE (DARK). *Cognitive functioning. Memory. Vascular functioning.* The cocoa that gives dark chocolate its haunting, addictive flavor is loaded with the memory-boosting antioxidant power of flavonoids. In two recent studies, cocoa consumption has been linked to higher scores on cognitive tests. Dark chocolate is also a boon to the cardiovascular system, and a healthy heart helps keep the brain sharp. Be warned, though: milk seems to interfere with the body's ability to access the power of flavonoids, so these benefits don't really apply to milk chocolate. And it might be best to steer clear of milk while you're enjoying that dark chocolate.

CILANTRO, CORIANDER. *Cognitive functioning. Memory.* Both of these spices come from the coriander plant, with the fresh leaves generally known as cilantro and the seeds generally know as coriander. They're popular in Asian, Indian, and Mexican cuisine. Cilantro and coriander have been shown to boost memory in mice. They also contain a good amount of vitamin K and a nice array of minerals that have been linked to healthier brain functioning.

CINNAMON. *Cognitive functioning. Focus. Memory. Neuronal health.* Scientists are finding intriguing connections between this ancient spice and the inner workings of the brain. Cinnamon delivers some anti-inflammatory benefits, which may well boost overall brain functioning. It also unleashes in the brain some special proteins called neurotrophic factors, which can help the brain generate new neurons and keep old ones healthy. Researchers also found that the sweet scent of cinnamon can improve memory and focus on cognitive tests. Interestingly, there's a compound called CEppt found in cinnamon bark, and the extract is now being studied for its potential in the fight against Alzheimer's disease.

COCONUT MILK. *Cognitive functioning. Focus. Mental energy. Mood.* Coconut milk is rich in unique substances called medium-chain triglycerides, which have been shown to improve cognitive performance in Alzheimer's patients after as little as a single serving. Plus, coconut milk is a great source of the key minerals we need to keep our minds sharp as we get older. And its thiamin and vitamin C can help maintain our energy and boost our mood.

CRANBERRIES. *Memory. Mood.* Cranberries are a great source of ursolic acid, which may have the potential to counteract some substances that can cause brain dysfunction. They also have good amounts of vitamin C, which can boost mood, and vitamin K, which may help memory. There's lots of antioxidant power in those two vitamins as well.

CUMIN. *Cognitive functioning. Learning.* This rich spice is loaded with iron, and iron deficiency ranks among the most common nutritional deficiencies in the world. Iron is especially important for women in their childbearing years, and it's been shown to boost brain performance in the eighteen-to-thirty-five set. Cumin is also a source of calcium and magnesium, a pair of minerals that may help prevent cognitive decline. Plus, cumin extract has been shown to boost learning skills in animal models.

EGGS. *Cognitive functioning. Focus. Memory.* There's quite a bit of the B vitamin choline in eggs, and that's good news for our brains. Choline has been shown to boost scores on cognitive tests and improve mental focus. Eggs also deliver healthy amounts of vitamin B_{12}, which has been linked with improved memory and a lower risk of cognitive decline later in life. The vitamin D in eggs may also help our brains stay healthy as we age.

FENNEL. *Cognitive functioning. Learning. Mood.* Fennel is a great source of the B vitamin folate, which has been shown to boost mental performance and may help prevent the onset of dementia. Vitamin C is also here in a good amount, and that, too, helps stave off mental decline. As a bonus, vitamin C can also help keep your spirits up. Finally, the vitamin A in fennel may deliver a boost to your learning abilities.

GARLIC. *Cognitive functioning. Memory.* No wonder garlic is one of the world's oldest cultivated plants—it's a boon to our overall health. It's been shown to boost memory and help keep our brains sharp later in life. It's also good for cardiovascular health, and that is strongly associated with better brain functioning. Perhaps most fascinating, garlic intake helps boost the body's iron metabolism, making it easier for that vital mineral to get to the places in the body where it needs to be. One of those places is the brain, as iron deficiencies are strongly linked with weaker cognitive performance.

GINGER. *Cognitive functioning. Focus. Memory.* Ginger is an antioxidant powerhouse, especially in the area of brain health. Many women can experience a loss of mental sharpness as they get into middle age, but ginger has been shown to help keep that from happening. Another study on postmenopausal women showed ginger boosting their memory skills and ability to focus. It's also been shown to boost memory after serious brain injuries.

GRAPEFRUIT. *Cognitive functioning. Learning. Mood.* Among the commonly available juices in grocery aisles, grapefruit ranks near the top when it comes to delivering the antioxidant goods. Whether as fruit or in juice, it's loaded with both vitamin C and vitamin A. The former has been shown to boost moods, while the latter has been linked with improved learning skills. Grapefruits are also great for cardiovascular health, something that is in turn associated with better cognitive functioning. Plus, fruit juices, including grapefruit juice, may help delay the onset of Alzheimer's in those most susceptible to the disease.

GREEN TEA. *Cognitive functioning. Focus. Memory. Neuronal health.* The antioxidants in green tea can really give your brain a lift. In studies, subjects who drank tea had more mental focus and better memory, with the latter result confirmed by MRI exams showing heightened activity in an area of the brain called the dorsolateral prefrontal cortex. Green tea has also been linked with helping the brain create new neurons. And a study of older Japanese found that those who drank more green tea in life had fewer cognitive impairments.

HALIBUT. *Cognitive functioning. Learning. Neuronal health.* Halibut is packed with nutrients that can help keep your brain performing at its best. There is vitamin D, which helps stave off cognitive decline as we get older. Vitamin A is here as well, and that seems to help regulate the brain's plasticity—its ability to form new neural pathways—and promote the ability to learn new mental skills. Halibut is also rich in omega-3 fatty acids, which may also protect against cognitive decline.

KALE. *Learning. Memory. Mood.* Put simply, kale is one of the healthiest foods you can eat. Packed with forty-five different varieties of antioxidant flavonoids, kale delivers

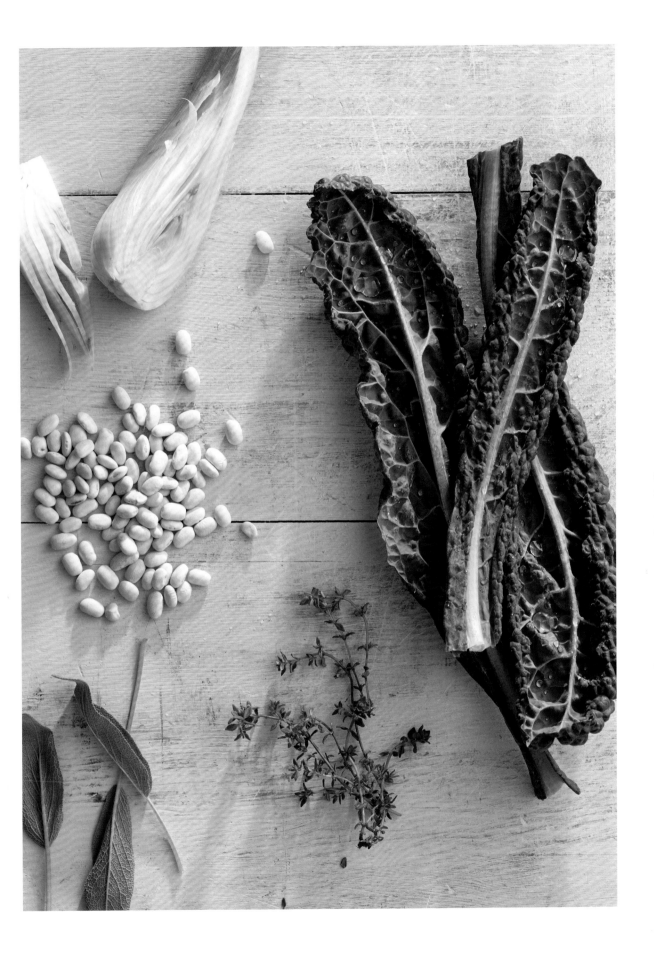

astounding amounts of vitamin K, which may boost our memories, and vitamin A, which can improve our learning skills. There's also a good amount of mood-elevating vitamin C in kale. Plus, it has important minerals that may well protect against cognitive decline.

LAMB. *Cognitive functioning. Focus. Memory. Mental energy. Mood. Neuronal health.* When talk turns to omega-3 fatty acids, most people think about fish. But lamb, too, delivers a healthy share of the acids that may help preserve the brain's plasticity and protect against cognitive decline. Lamb is also a strong source of vitamin B_{12}, which has been linked with better memory and less depression. Another B vitamin, niacin, is here as well, and it has been associated with improved mental energy and the prevention of cognitive decline. Lamb is also a great source of zinc, which may well boost memory functioning.

LEEKS. *Cognitive functioning. Focus. Learning. Memory. Neuronal health.* Like fellow alliums onions and garlic, leeks are perhaps best known for their ability to deliver cardiovascular benefits, which lead in turn to higher cognitive functioning. Leeks are also a good source of vitamin K, which can improve memory, and vitamin A, which can boost learning skills and help the brain maintain its plasticity. Important B vitamins are here as well, including B_6, which helps in focus and attention, and folate, which may protect against long-term cognitive decline.

LEGUMES (BEANS, LENTILS, AND PEAS). *Cognitive functioning. Memory. Mental energy.* Regular consumption of beans, peas, and lentils will help keep your brain sharp and healthy. A large study in China found that older people who consumed beans, peas, and lentils more often were less likely to be suffering from cognitive decline. Legumes are also loaded with B vitamins like thiamin, riboflavin, and niacin. These have been linked with sharper mental focus, less fatigue, and better memory, respectively. Legumes are also rich in key minerals that can help keep the mind sharp and the brain healthy.

LEMONS AND LIMES. *Cognitive functioning. Memory. Mood.* These two fruits are veritable vitamin C factories. A powerful antioxidant, vitamin C has been linked with better brain health in older people and happier moods. Lemons and limes are also loaded with memory-boosting flavonoids. And the folate they provide may protect against cognitive decline.

LENTILS. *Cognitive functioning. Focus. Memory.* Lentils are full of the brain-friendly B vitamins. Their folate helps keep our minds sharp as we age. Their thiamin and vitamin B_6 help give us more focus and energy. They're a good source of iron, which is vitally important to cognitive functioning during a woman's childbearing years. And they're a good source of a potential memory-booster, zinc.

MINT. *Cognitive functioning. Focus. Learning. Memory. Neuronal health.* Some of mint's effects on the brain come from nutrients. It's a good source of vitamin A, which can help boost learning skills and increase the brain's plasticity. There's some vitamin C in mint as well, which may protect against cognitive decline. But there are also fascinating studies out there about how the scent of mint affects brain functioning. In one study, the aroma of mint helped boost alertness and memory. In another, it helped test subjects perform better on basic clerical skills, such as typing and memorization.

MUSHROOMS. *Cognitive functioning. Focus. Mental energy. Memory.* Mushrooms are another of those vitamin B powerhouses that need be a regular part of your brain-healthy diet. Vitamin B2, or riboflavin, is here to help reduce fatigue. Vitamin B6 improves your mental focus. Vitamin B3, or niacin, assists your memory and boosts energy levels. Mushrooms are also a pretty good source of vitamin D, which may well help protect against long-term cognitive decline.

OATS. *Cognitive functioning. Focus. Healthy sleep. Learning. Mental energy.* Oats are most famous for being amazingly heart-healthy, but that, too, affects your brain for the better. A recent study found that people at risk for heart disease scored significantly worse on cognitive tests than people with a healthier cardiovascular system. The differences started to appear as early as age thirty-five. Oats also boost the brain directly. Studies in children show that oatmeal is the best breakfast if you're looking for mentally productive mornings. Oats are also a good source of thiamin, which can boost our concentration levels and give us more mental energy. They also have magnesium, which can help with our memory, our learning skills, and our sleeping habits.

OLIVE OIL. *Cognitive functioning. Memory.* Extra-virgin olive oil is chock-full of "good fats." Some 75 percent of its fats come in the form of the monounsaturated oleic acid—more than any other oil. Studies have shown that olive oil consumption is associated with a stronger memory and higher scores on verbal fluency tests. Those "good fats" have been linked in studies to improved memory and better overall brain functioning. Olive oil is also renowned as a key element in a heart-healthy diet, and cardiovascular health is strongly related to better cognitive functioning.

OLIVES. *Cognitive functioning. Learning. Neuronal health.* Whether black, green, or kalamata style, olives are good for the brain. They have lots of vitamin A, which has been linked with improvements in learning capabilities and in the plasticity of the brain. Vitamin E can help prevent mental decline as we get older. Olives are also a good source of iron, and iron deficiencies are associated with cognitive problems, both in older people and in women of childbearing age.

ONIONS. *Cognitive functioning. Energy. Focus. Memory. Neuronal health.* Onions are a rich source of antioxidant flavonoids, but remember that much of that power is concentrated in the outer parts of the onions so you shouldn't overpeel them. Those flavonoids have been shown to boost memory and protect neurons from injury. One study found that onions had neuroprotective qualities that reduced the chance of strokes. In animal models, it's been shown that onions can help combat depression. They're also a good source of a couple of the B vitamins, including thiamin, which is linked to more mental focus and higher energy levels.

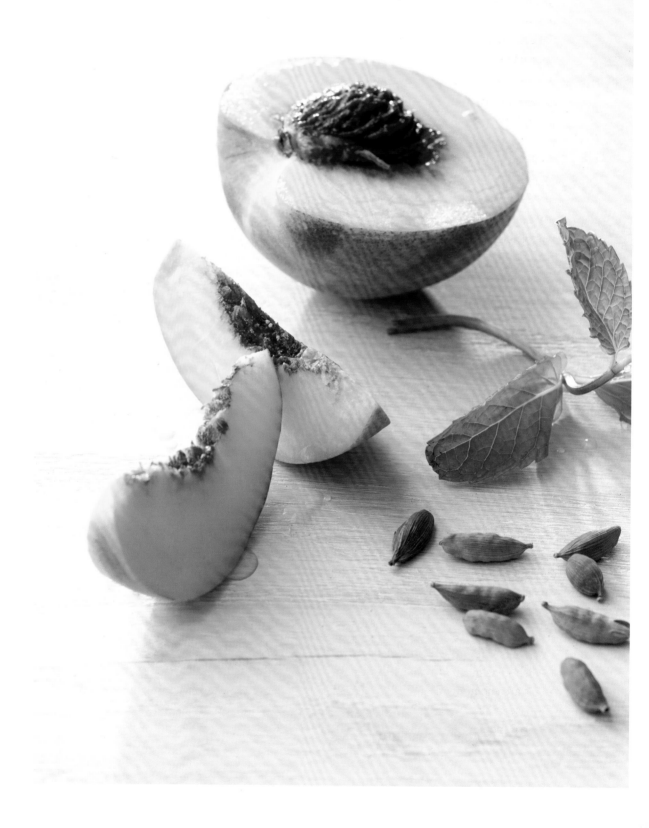

ORANGES. *Cognitive functioning. Learning. Memory. Mood. Neuronal health.* An antioxidant powerhouse, oranges boast more than 170 different kinds of phytonutrients and more than 60 different flavonoids. That's good news for your memory and overall brain health. Oranges are loaded with vitamin C, which can help boost your mood. There's also a good amount of vitamin A in oranges, which could help improve your learning skills and enhance brain plasticity.

OREGANO. *Cognitive functioning. Healthy sleep. Memory. Mood. Motivation.* A staple spice in Mediterranean and Mexican dishes, oregano is an excellent source of vitamin K, linked with both overall cognitive health and improved memory. There's iron in oregano, too, and iron deficiencies are strongly associated with cognitive problems. Scientists are now looking at connections between oregano extracts and cognitive function, with two recent studies in animal models showing beneficial effects on mood, motivation, and sleeping patterns.

PARSLEY. *Cognitive functioning. Learning. Memory.* Parsley is loaded with a powerful flavonoid called luteolin that's been linked with memory improvements. Its also got lots of vitamin A, which can help boost learning skills as well as maintain overall brain health. Vitamin K is here in good measure as well, and that can help keep our brains sharp.

PARSNIPS. *Cognitive functioning. Focus. Mood.* Parsnips are a solid source of the antioxidant powerhouse vitamin C, which can boost mood and help keep your brain in top shape as you age. The B vitamins folate and choline are here in good amounts, too. Choline has been linked with stronger mental focus and better performance on cognitive tests. Folate may help prevent dementia later in life.

PEACHES. *Cognitive functioning. Focus. Learning. Memory. Mental energy. Mood.* Peaches are a sweet source of a trio of brain-boosting vitamins. Vitamin C can lift your mood; vitamin K can help your memory; and vitamin A can improve your learning skills. There's a good amount of the B vitamin niacin in peaches as well. That may help give you more mental energy. Peaches also deliver a trio of key minerals—potassium, calcium, and magnesium—that may help slow cognitive decline and prevent strokes.

PISTACHIOS. *Cognitive functioning. Focus. Memory. Mental energy.* This member of the cashew family may be able to help you find more mental focus and energy, as it contains a wealth of the B vitamin thiamin. Vitamin K is here in good measure as well, and that's good news for your memory and long-term cognitive health. The folate in pistachios may also help prevent dementia, and the zinc they hold may help ward off depression.

POMEGRANATES. *Cognitive functioning. Memory. Mood.* Because pomegranates contain unusually high levels of antioxidant polyphenols, they are often dubbed one of the "superfruits." In recent years, scientists have started looking at whether pomegranates and their juice might help in the fight against Alzheimer's disease. Initial results in animal models are encouraging. Another recent study found that pomegranate juice prevented the otherwise natural lapses in memory that occur in the months after heart surgery. Rich in vitamin C, pomegranates might also help boost your moods. They also deliver quite a bit of vitamin K and the B vitamin folate, both of which have been shown to protect against the loss of brain function in our later years.

POTATOES. *Cognitive functioning. Focus. Memory. Mood.* When faced with a cognitive challenge, many people look to protein for mental fuel. But the carbohydrates in potatoes may be able to do the trick as well. In one recent study, subjects who ate potatoes did much better on cognitive tests than others. Potatoes are also a good source of vitamin B6, which may be able to help sharpen our mental focus. There's a lot of vitamin C in potatoes as well, and that can help us stay in productive moods. The same vitamin C might also protect against long-term cognitive decline.

PUMPKIN. *Cognitive functioning. Learning. Mood. Mental energy. Neuronal health.* Pumpkins aren't just for carving on Halloween. They're also a great source of the powerful vitamin A, which can boost the plasticity of the brain and may also help make it easier to learn new mental skills. The riboflavin in pumpkin has been shown to raise cognitive-skill test scores in young people. Pumpkins also deliver the antioxidant vitamins A and C, which can protect against long-term cognitive decline.

PUMPKIN SEEDS. *Cognitive functioning. Learning. Memory. Mood.* They may be tiny little things, but pumpkins seeds, aka pepitas, pack a brain-healthy punch. They're loaded with zinc, for starters, and zinc deficiency can be a problem in Western diets. Recent studies show zinc helping to improve our memories and keep depression at bay. Pumpkin seeds are a good source of iron as well, and iron deficiency is one of the more common nutritional problems in the world. Especially in women of childbearing years, iron has been shown to boost cognitive performance. Pumpkin seeds also deliver generous helpings of a mineral trio—potassium, magnesium, and calcium—that's been shown to delay cognitive decline.

QUINOA. *Cognitive functioning. Memory. Mood.* This tiny seed, which humans in the Andes have been cultivating for 4,000 years, is rich in nutrients and generally regarded as even more heart-healthy than cereal grasses such as wheat. That's great for the brain, too, as our cardiac health is closely linked with our cognitive health, starting as early as our mid-thirties. Quinoa is also a good source of zinc, which can be hard to get in Western diets. Zinc helps keep our memory strong, and it may help stave off depression. There's a lot of folate here as well, and that's a B vitamin that promotes brain health as we age, possibly even helping to prevent dementia.

RAISINS. *Cognitive functioning. Focus. Memory. Mental energy.* One of the most convenient snacks available also delivers healthy helpings of two minerals that keep your brain sharp. It's a challenge to get boron through the diet, but the brain and body need it to convert estrogen and vitamin D to their most active forms. Whether you get enough boron may end up affecting your memory, your focus, and even your eye-hand coordination, and raisins can help. The other mineral in raisins is iron, and iron deficiencies can cause cognitive problems, especially in women during the childbearing years. Raisins also have the B vitamin thiamin, which has been linked with getting more mental focus and energy. Another B vitamin in raisins, choline, has been linked with better overall cognitive functioning.

RASPBERRIES. *Cognitive functioning. Memory. Mood.* One recent study of people who ate lots of berries found that they maintained their cognitive functioning an extra two years compared with nonberry eaters. Raspberries deliver lots of mood-elevating vitamin C and memory-boosting vitamin K. They also have good amounts of vitamin E and the B vitamin folate, both of which have been linked with stronger cognitive performance.

ROSEMARY. *Cognitive functioning. Learning. Memory. Mood.* Two recent studies have linked this herb with better brain functioning. In one, subjects who consumed rosemary showed stronger memory skills. In the other, the focus was on the scent of rosemary, which helped subjects boost their speed and accuracy on various cognitive tasks. Rosemary is a great source of vitamin A, which may help boost learning skills, and of vitamin C, which can elevate your moods. Rosemary is also rich in the minerals zinc and iron. The former is a memory booster and may help keep depression at bay, while the latter is especially important to the cognitive function of women in the childbearing years.

SAFFRON. *Cognitive functioning. Healthy sleep. Learning. Memory. Mood.* In one recent study, this exotic spice seemed to help Alzheimer's patients do better on cognitive tests. It's also been shown to boost memory in tests with animals. Saffron is a great source of iron, and iron deficiencies can cause a number of different cognitive problems, especially in women during their childbearing years. Saffron also has healthy amounts of magnesium, which has been linked to better sleeping habits and improved learning skills. Vitamin C, a mood booster, and vitamin A, which may also help boost learning skills, are in saffron as well.

SAGE. *Cognitive functioning. Focus. Healthy sleep. Learning. Memory.* For centuries, herbalists have used this member of the mint family as a memory aid. Researchers investigated further, and they found that subjects given sage oil did indeed score much better on memory tests. Sage is packed with the memory-booster vitamin K, as well as with vitamin A, which is linked with improvements in learning skills. There's thiamin here, too, to improve mental focus. On the mineral side, sage is a wonderful source of the iron we need to maintain our cognitive health and the magnesium that may help us sleep better.

SALMON (WILD). *Cognitive functioning. Focus. Mental energy.* The consumption of fish rich in omega-3 fatty acids has been linked in several studies with stronger cognitive performance—both in middle age and in our older years. Wild salmon is also a good source of niacin, which may help with your mental energy, and of choline, which may help strengthen your mental focus.

SARDINES. *Cognitive functioning. Memory. Mental energy. Mood.* This oily fish is loaded with the brain-boosting vitamin B_{12}, which may boost our memories and help ward off depression. Sardines are a rich source of the omega-3 fatty acids that help keep our brains sharper as we get into middle age and beyond. There's a lot of niacin in sardines as well, and that may help us find more mental energy.

SCALLOPS. *Cognitive functioning. Focus. Healthy sleep. Learning. Memory.* Scallops are loaded with vitamin B12, which has been linked with memory gains and with maintaining overall brain functioning. There's also a good amount of choline here, which may help sharpen your mental focus. Scallops are a good source of minerals, too. They've got zinc, which may help stave off depression, and magnesium, which promotes learning skills and healthy sleeping patterns.

SESAME SEEDS. *Cognitive functioning. Healthy sleep. Memory.* Sesame seeds are a treasure trove of key minerals. They're a great source of zinc, which may help prevent depression and improve memory. There's a lot of magnesium here as well, which may be good for our memory, our learning skills, and our sleeping habits. Plus, sesame seeds have iron, and steering clear of iron deficiencies is essential to brain health.

SHRIMP. *Cognitive functioning. Focus. Learning. Memory. Mood.* Shrimp doesn't have as much of the brain-boosting omega-3 fatty acids as we've seen in other seafood, but it still has a good amount. It's also loaded with vitamin B12, which may help improve your memory and reduce the risk you'll suffer from depression. The choline and B6 in shrimp may help you focus more on mental tasks, and the zinc here is important to the functioning of our memories.

SQUASH. *Cognitive functioning. Focus. Learning. Memory. Neuronal health.* Generally speaking, the winter squashes pack more of a nutritional punch than the summer ones, but both will help keep your brain healthy and your mind sharp. There's lots of vitamin A in squash, which boosts the plasticity of the brain and may help improve our learning skills. The vitamin C here may help to keep bad moods away, while the vitamin B6 helps us concentrate more. There's a decent amount of vitamin K in squash as well, and that's good news for our memories.

STRAWBERRIES. *Cognitive functioning. Healthy sleep. Memory. Mood.* In recent studies, berry consumption has been linked to the prevention of brain damage and to delays in cognitive decline as we get up there in years. There's a good amount of vitamin C in strawberries, which can help keep our moods up. The folate here helps keep our brains sharp as we age. And strawberries have magnesium, too. That mineral can help our memories and sleeping patterns.

SUNFLOWER SEEDS. *Cognitive functioning. Mental energy.* One the oldest cultivated seeds— Native Americans have grown sunflowers for more than 5,000 years—sunflower seeds are a warehouse of several important vitamins and minerals. Their high vitamin E content has been linked to a reduction of inflammation and cognitive decline, while their vitamin B1 (thiamin) stores may boost energy. Sunflower seeds are also rich in magnesium, linked to a lower risk of stroke and migraines.

SWEET POTATOES. *Cognitive functioning. Focus. Learning. Mental energy. Neuronal health.* In Africa, where vitamin A deficiency can be a serious problem, scientists have learned that sweet potatoes can make a world of difference. They are positively loaded with beta-carotene, which the body converts into vitamin A. And vitamin A, in turn, can help improve our learning skills and boost the brain's plasticity. Several B vitamins are in sweet potatoes as well, including B6, niacin, and B1—all of which can help sharpen our mental focus and concentration. And you might want to keep an eye out for purple sweet potatoes. A recent study found indications that they may be especially good at preventing cognitive problems.

SWISS CHARD. *Cognitive functioning. Healthy sleep. Learning. Memory.* This leafy green vegetable is a great source of memory-boosting vitamin K. It's also loaded with vitamin A, which has been linked with improvements in various learning skills. The array of B vitamins here, including folate and B6, may help keep the brain healthier and sharper as we age. Swiss chard also contains the minerals iron and zinc. Avoiding iron deficiencies is critical to avoiding cognitive complications in life. And zinc boosts our memories and may help keep depression at bay.

THYME. *Cognitive functioning. Learning. Mood. Neuronal health.* Thyme contains a pair of brain-boosting vitamins, A and C. Vitamin A can help maintain the health of our brains over the long haul of life. It's also linked with improved learning skills and more plasticity in our brains. Vitamin C, too, may help the brain stay sharp over the course of our lives. It can also boost our moods. There's some iron in thyme as well, and iron deficiencies are associated with numerous cognitive problems.

TOMATOES. *Cognitive functioning. Focus. Learning. Memory. Neuronal health. Vascular health.* The tomato is best known in nutrition circles for its benefits to our cardiovascular health. Those benefits pay off in the brain as well, as people with low risk factors for heart disease score higher on cognitive tests. Tomatoes are a great source of vitamin A, which builds our brain's plasticity and may help improve our learning skills. Memory-boosting vitamin K is here as well. And tomatoes deliver a bevy of B vitamins—folate, niacin, B6—that are associated with stronger mental focus, energy, and better long-term cognitive function. The antioxidant lycopene, high in tomatoes, has been associated with potential protective benefits against Parkinson's disease. Tomatoes, especially those used in sauces where their fibers have been broken down, may help offset lycopene deficiencies that have been found in investigations into Alzheimer's disease, mild cognitive impairments, and vascular dementia.

TUNA. *Cognitive functioning. Focus. Memory. Mood.* Tuna is a great source for an amazing five different B vitamins that are good for the brain. Niacin and vitamin B12 may help improve our memories. Choline, vitamin B6, and vitamin B1 can help sharpen our mental focus and give us more mental energy. Tuna is also a great source of the omega-3 fatty acids, which can boost our overall cognitive performance while also helping to ease anxiety. There's some vitamin D in tuna, too, and that may help slow cognitive decline as we get older.

TURKEY. *Cognitive functioning. Focus. Memory. Mood.* The best choice here is pasture-raised turkey, as the meat from those birds are likely to contain more protein and a better ratio of good fats like the omega-3 fatty acids to bad ones. Turkey is a strong source of all the B vitamins, including three—niacin, B6, and choline—that can improve our mental energy and focus. Vitamin B12 is here, too, and that's a memory booster. It has also been linked with reducing the risk of cognitive decline as we get older. Turkey is also a good source of zinc, which may help keep depression at bay while also helping our memories.

TURMERIC. *Cognitive functioning. Focus. Vascular health.* The substance that gives turmeric its unique yellow-orange color is called curcumin, and it's gaining more attention among scientists lately. In animal models, it's been shown to boost cognitive functioning, especially in older subjects. It's also been shown in animals to protect against cardiovascular problems, which in turn can help to keep our brains sharp and healthy. There's also a good amount of iron in turmeric, and we need to stay away from iron deficiencies to protect the health of our brain. Turmeric is also a good source of vitamin B6, which can help improve our mental focus.

WALNUTS. *Cognitive functioning. Focus. Healthy sleep. Memory. Vascular health.* When using walnuts, it's best to leave the skins on, as that's where most of this tree nut's powerful antioxidant phenols reside. A number of studies in recent years have turned up evidence that walnuts can help keep your cardiovascular system healthy. That's important to the brain, too, as researchers have found that people with low risk factors for heart disease do better on cognitive tests. Studies in animal models have shown that walnuts may be able to boost cognitive functioning by working directly in the brain as well. There are important B vitamins here, including thiamin and B6. Both are linked with improved levels of concentration and mental energy. Walnuts also boast good amounts of zinc, a memory booster, and magnesium, which may help better regulate our sleeping patterns.

YOGURT. *Cognitive functioning. Memory. Mood.* Yogurt has been linked with memory improvements, as well as with helping to boost scores on cognitive tests taken by college students who had yogurt as a midafternoon snack. Yogurt is also an excellent source of zinc, which has been linked with improvements in memory and keeping depression at bay. The vitamin B12 in yogurt is good for the long term—it can help slow the process of cognitive decline in our later years.

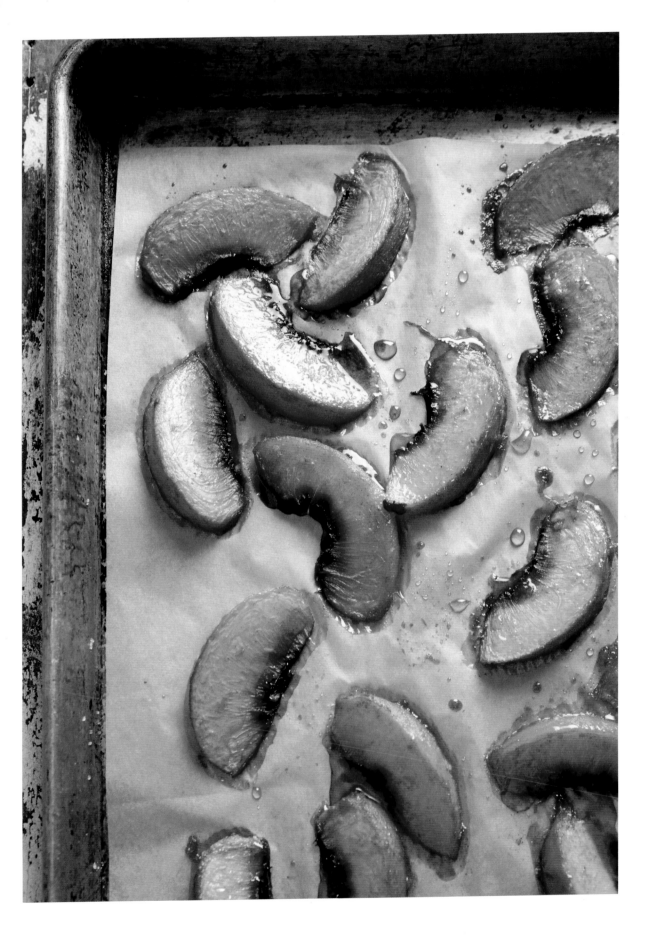

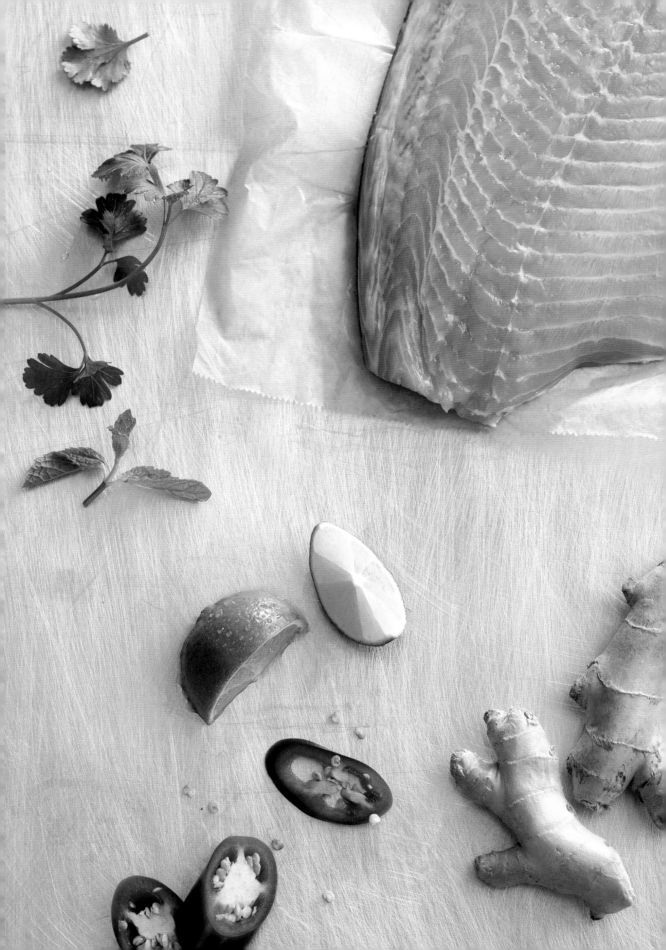

CHAPTER 3

Building Mind-Blowing Taste and Flavor

IF THERE'S ONE QUESTION I get time and again when I'm teaching people to cook, it's this: "How can healthy food taste great?"

Now, I'm not sure why that question is foremost in people's minds, though it's certainly reflective of a conundrum deep-seated in the American psyche, a myth promoted by well-meaning parents during our childhoods ("If you don't eat your veggies, no dessert!") and marketed by manufacturers of seemingly more exciting junk foods, but no matter . . . I'm here to not only tell you the truth, but *show* you the truth:

Great, brain-boosting foods taste *fantastic*.

All they need is a little love, and I have just the simple tool that provides all that and more. It's called FASS—which stands for fat, acid, salt, and sweet. By using basic pantry staples—olive oil (fat), lemon (acid), sea salt (salt), and Grade B organic maple syrup (sweet)—you can, just as cooks have been doing for centuries, learn to perfectly balance the five known tastes (salt, sweet, sour, bitter, and savory) in any dish.

I'll explain how in a moment, but first, let's look at your taste buds and taste in general. Both are fascinating topics, and appropriate for a brain book since all taste sensors lead, directly or indirectly, to the brain. I say indirectly because—get this—there are taste buds *throughout the body*. A story published in the journal *Nature* noted there are taste buds to be found in the gut, pancreas, lungs—even in sperm.

While we don't know the function of all of these below-the-throat taste buds, there have been some spectacular discoveries. Sugar, for example, receives a so-called "second tasting" in the gut. The taste bud receptors there, when they sense sugar, set off the release of glucose (aka sugar) into the cells. In turn, that releases insulin into the bloodstream to control sugar metabolism. From a culinary and physiological viewpoint, what's important to note is that artificial sweeteners also set off this reaction in the stomach, despite their reputation for not inducing "sugarlike" reactions anywhere other than the taste buds of the mouth. So that diet soda is hitting your gut as if it were the real deal.

How does this affect the brain? A couple of ways. Keeping blood sugar low may be important for everyone, not just diabetics or people with insulin resistance (aka pre-diabetics). A 2013 study published in *Neurology* found people with consistently lower blood sugar levels did better on memory tests. Conversely, higher blood sugar levels made the proteins in the brain associated with Alzheimer's disease more toxic. It used to be thought that the presence of the proteins themselves (called beta-amyloid proteins) were responsible for dementia; now the focus is shifting to the damage beta-amyloids cause to the blood vessels of the brain in the presence of high blood sugar.

One thing that's clear: the brain wants to know what it's tasting. In fact, it has backups for backups to make sure it doesn't miss a single molecule of taste. Consider that researchers estimate we have anywhere from 5,000 to 10,000 taste buds in and around our mouths, mostly on the top of the tongue but also underneath and on the roof of the mouth. There are up to a hundred taste receptors on each bud, so it's thought that each bud can sense a wide variety of tastes. There are also three major nerve "roadways" that each are capable of delivering taste sensation to the brain.

That's just the delivery system. On the receiving end, scientists have found unique areas in the brain that correspond to tastes such as salt and sweet and savory—or, as the Japanese call savory, "umami." It's possible, even probable, that the brain separates tastes to different regions for a reason; for example, bitterness, which from a survival viewpoint often meant poison, may relate to the part of the brain that deals with aversion—as in "avoid at all costs"—while sweet may be hardwired to sections of the brain devoted to cravings and the need for energy.

But taste is just one part of the equation. The other is smell, which when combined with taste is thought to create the perception of flavor. (If you don't believe this, consider the last time you had a serious cold that clogged up your nose. Betcha food was flavorless, yes?)

When hunger occurs, the brain sends a signal to the olfactory (smell) bulb located right behind the nose, essentially cranking up our ability to smell food. Scientists long wondered what the receptors for smell were; turns out they're part of the brain's endocannabinoid system (don't try pronouncing it; you'll only twist your tongue). Why is that cool? Because the same system in the brain is tied into memory and emotion. So all that talk about food = love and feeling good (I like looking at the positive emotions) isn't just talk; it's science. And the next time a real estate agent has chocolate chip cookies baking in the oven of an open house, you'll realize it's the cookies you love, not necessarily the house.

So now that we've hashed out smell and taste and flavor, the trick is making it all work for you in the kitchen. That's where FASS (remember FASS?) comes in. FASS acts like a culinary compass, allowing you to hone in on the exact taste you're looking for by manipulating a meal's fat, acid, salt, and sweet content. Those four factors are what

I call taste and flavor carriers, so let's take a moment to consider each of these players and what they bring to the pot and the plate.

- FAT (OLIVE OIL): Fats serve several purposes. Think of fats as waves on which all the tastes surf. Fat becomes the transport mechanism carrying tastes all over the mouth and across the taste buds. That's vital, especially as we age and the sensitivity of our taste buds begins to wane. Fat also satiates; without it in a dish, you'd never feel full. It slows down the release of sugars into the bloodstream. And it increases the bioavailability of fat-soluble vitamins in other foods.

- ACID (LEMON JUICE): Acids make food pop, brightening any dish. They also act as the starting gun for your salivary glands, calling them to action, which improves your digestion. As with fats, acids also reduce the rate at which sugar is released into the bloodstream, lowering the glycemic load.

- SALT (SEA SALT): From a cooking perspective, salt serves a vital purpose: it breaks down fibers, notably in vegetables, releasing the inherent taste of a food (that's why, if you want a veggie to release its natural sweetness, you have to use a bit of salt). On the palate, salt gives the perception of taste moving toward the front of the mouth.

- SWEET (MAPLE SYRUP): Sweet is a natural counterbalance to sour and has the ability to tame a dish down if it's become too spicy (see the chart FASS Fixes in the Kitchen on page 31).

Why these foods? I'm glad you asked. Not all FASS is created equal. There's good FASS—the foods I use, which nourish the brain—and bad FASS, which is what you'll often find in processed foods and which isn't good for the brain or the body. There's a chart of good and bad FASS (see page 32), but for now let's look at the good FASS.

For oil, I always prefer extra-virgin olive oil. It's the staple of the Mediterranean diet and it may be, in large part, why there's such longevity in that area of the world. Extra-virgin olive oil is the least processed of the olive oils, has a great ratio of monounsaturated to saturated fat, and has anti-inflammatory and anticoagulation properties.

For acid, I stick to lemon juice or a close citrus cousin such as lime or orange. These flavors aren't overpowering, as is vinegar, but really allow me to add a little pizzazz to a dish that otherwise might be blah.

With salt, I always, always, always use sea salt. Unlike bleached, refined table salt, sea salt has nearly eighty different minerals.

As for sweet, I primarily go with Grade B organic maple syrup. I know that's a surprise to some people, but it's a lot healthier (notably rich in zinc and manganese) than refined sugar and far mellower and more full-bodied, meaning a little goes a long way.

FASS in Action

Cooking is as much a head game as anything else. I've seen many people come into the kitchen for the first time, and for lack of a better phrase, they're already psyched out. They've convinced themselves that if they make one wrong move they'll wreck the dish. That leads to culinary paralysis-by-analysis, sort of like an ice skater who is so worried about taking a tumble that he ties himself in knots throughout his performance. To be able to flow freely and beautifully—whether in the rink or the kitchen—you *must* give yourself permission to be fully present and responsive to changes as they occur.

The best way I know how to teach people to be present is to cook up a pot of soup. There's something about starting with water and adding ingredients one by one that pulls them in, as the heat from the flame begins to work its magic on the elements in the pot. As the smells begin wafting up, there's something almost hypnotic taking place; you can see people want to taste what's going on, but they're hesitant, like a kid wondering whether she can step into her father's workshop when Dad isn't present.

I say, step right in and taste, taste, taste! That's what cooking, *real* cooking is all about, knowing that you're in charge of the taste, as opposed to the taste being in charge of you. As a tool, FASS is the great fixer, a culinary Swiss Army knife that allows you to adjust flavor on the fly.

What's this mean in the real world? Let's go back to the soup example. Often, as the soup builds, I'll purposely throw off the flavor by, say, adding too much salt. I'll then invite my students to come up and taste the soup. They'll make the inevitable stinky face, and you can see the words form in their mind—*This soup is ruined. It'll have to be tossed.*

Ah, but no. The soup isn't toast, it's just out of balance. If you're old enough to remember analog car radios, you know that the station would sometimes drift, but you could fine-tune it and knock out all the static with just a slight turn of the dial. Similarly, it's easy to rebalance a dish and make it sing true by using a FASS fix. In the example I just gave, all it takes is a spritz of lemon to neutralize the oversalting. What's amazing is seeing the look on a person's face when they employ FASS, take a quick taste, and realize they've not only avoided a culinary disaster, but also brought a dish back into perfect form.

Nearly anything that goes wrong with a dish—too bitter, too salty, too sour—can be fixed by FASS, but FASS isn't only about rectifying mistakes. It's also the way to, as I say, take a good-tasting meal completely over the top. FASS can act as the perfect finishing agent, the proverbial cherry on top of the sundae. I can't tell you the number of times I've had people taste a dish and say, "Hey, that's good," to which I reply, "Okay, fine, but what do we have to do to take it to 'yum!'?" What's wonderful, and, I think, innate within the brain, is the ability to access and articulate what taste is missing to hit that "yum" button. With a certain amount of practice, I've seen even kitchen newbies verbalize what FASS factor needs to be tweaked to reach yum, and when it happens you can see their confidence blossom.

To me, the fun part about FASS is its simplicity. I've had colleagues taste a dish I've made and say, "Wow, that's really seasoned well! What did you use?" When I tell them, they're like, "You only used lemon?!" They're expecting some exotic spice, and while I do use spices and herbs extensively (see Spicy Solutions, page 33), FASS is as easy to use as lemon or, say, a drape of mape (as in maple syrup).

FASS is a starting point for culinary creativity. As you gain more confidence, you'll find you can expand on the basic flavor carriers. In this book, for example, I've gone beyond olive oil at times when it comes to including a healthy fat. I may use ghee (clarified butter), or a nut cream such as walnut or cashew cream, or an avocado. For an acid, instead of reaching for a lemon, I might choose a balsamic or rice vinegar, or use sauerkraut in a dish. For sweet, there's raisins and dates, or a caramelized onion or roasted tomato.

The point is, once you realize you need a certain flavor carrier, there are plenty of healthy, delicious, delightful options out there. FASS will get you started; where you finish is limited only by your imagination.

FASS FOR FLAVOR AND BRAIN HEALTH

	EXAMPLES	FUNCTION	HEALTH BENEFITS
FAT	avocado, butter, coconut oil, ghee, nuts, olive oil, sesame oil	Distributes flavor across the palate.	Increases satiety. Makes foods high in brain boosting fat-soluble vitamins more bioavailable.
ACID	lemons, limes, orange, vinegar	Brightens flavors.	Increases absorption of brain-boosting minerals and stimulates digestion.
SALT	sea salt	Brings out the flavor of foods. Moves flavor to the front of the tongue where it's best perceived.	In balance with potassium, facilitates energy production and cellular metabolism.
SWEET	dates, grade b maple syrup, honey, blackstrap molasses, raisins	Tames harsh, sour, or spicy flavors. Rounds out or harmonizes flavors.	Increases sense of pleasure.

FASS FIXES IN THE KITCHEN

PROBLEM	FASS FIX
Too sweet?	Add lemon juice or another acid.
Too sour?	Add maple syrup or another sweetener.
Too bland?	Add salt.
Too salty?	Add lemon juice or another acid, which will erase the taste of salt.
Just needs a spark?	Add fresh lemon or lime at the end of cooking.
Too harsh?	Add $1/8$ to $1/4$ teaspoon Grade B maple syrup.

NATURAL VERSUS PROCESSED FASS

	NATURAL: BRAIN BOOSTING	PROCESSED: BRAIN ZAPPING
FATS	• butter • coconut oil • ghee • grapeseed oil • extra-virgin olive oil • sesame oil	• corn oil • cottonseed oil • elaidic acid (trans fat) • interesterified fat (industrially produced/unnatural) • saturated fats that replace trans fats • meat and egg products (factory-farmed) • partially hydrogenated vegetable oils • soybean oil
ACIDS	• grapefruit • lemons • limes • oranges • organic vinegars	• artificial food colorings and preservatives • benzoic acid (used as a preservative) • citric acid (not bad if naturally occurring, but artificially produced 330 and E330 citric acid additives are made using sulfuric acid and may contain sulfites and mold not filtered out in production, causing asthma and hyperactivity)
SALT	• kosher salt • sea salt	• autolyzed yeast extract (flavor enhancer and source of hidden gluten) • disodium guanylate • disodium inosinate • monosodium glutamate (MSG) • sodium benzoate • sodium bisulfite • sodium nitrate • sodium saccharin • sulfur dioxide
SUGARS	• grade b maple syrup • honey • blackstrap molasses	• acesulfame potassium • aspartame and other artificial sugars • corn syrup • cyclamate and cyclamic acid • dextrin • dextrose • fructose • high-fructose corn syrup • maltodextrin • saccharin • refined white sugar

The Fifth Taste: Umami

Settling a long-lasting controversy, scientists and gourmands have finally come to an agreement over the last few years that umami is indeed a basic taste—perhaps *the* way we taste amino acids (aka proteins). The word *umami* is Japanese for "savory," and it's used to describe how certain foods lend a (pick one) meatiness, brothiness, weight, or gravity to a dish.

Scientists find umami fascinating because it appears to be sensed by the parts of the taste buds that pick up glutamate (if that sounds familiar, it's because monosodium glutamate (MSG) is an artificial flavor enhancer that imparts umami, most notoriously in Chinese-restaurant food). Glutamate has an important role as a neurotransmitter; not only does it appear to play a part in memory and learning, but in digestion as well. There are glutamate receptors in the stomach, and it's thought that when you eat a food with glutamate, a signal goes through the glutamate receptors along the vagus nerve to the brain that it's time for digestion to begin.

When you're looking to introduce umami into something you're cooking, you're in luck; there are a surprising number of foods that can impart that savory feel, that sensation of heft and heartiness. These include tomatoes, sweet potatoes, anchovies, and more (see list, below).

For my money, umami-rich foods are major flavor boosters, which is why many of them are in the recipes in this book. They add a must-have dimension to a meal's taste and texture. Whenever you can get an umami food into the mix, go for it!

UMAMI-RICH FOODS

VEGETABLES: Carrots, mushrooms, potatoes, sweet potatoes, tomatoes

MEAT: beef, chicken, lamb

SEAFOOD: anchovies, cod, kombu, sardines, scallops, shrimp

CONDIMENTS: fish sauce, tomato paste

OTHER: Parmesan cheese, green tea, red wine

Spicy Solutions

Cooking is a little bit like working out: keep your workout routine the same and pretty soon the body gets used to it and plateaus instead of getting stronger. Similarly, taste buds fed the same food day after day will fatigue; what once was a striking, stimulating taste will no longer trigger that same intensely pleasurable response.

What you need are new stimuli to throw your taste buds a curveball and keep them engaged. Where you'll find something new is in the use of herbs and spices. From a brain health perspective, many herbs and spices, teaspoon for teaspoon, contain huge amounts of anti-inflammatories and antioxidants, as a quick review of the Culinary Pharmacy (page 9) will reveal. If we're talking taste, their influence is just as powerful on both the mouth and the nose. Recall that flavor is the combination of both the sense of smell and the sense of taste; nothing turns that on more than the so-called aromatics: herbs, spices, and members of the allium family including leeks, garlic, shallots, onions, and chives.

Another interesting aspect of herbs and spices is that they invigorate both appetite and satiation. So you'll want to eat as soon as the first hint of spice hits your nose, and you'll dive in with taste buds energized to the max, but you'll also step away from the table sooner (and happier) than if you hadn't employed herbs and spices. If you're new to the aromatics game, fret not; see the chart below for a comprehensive list of global flavorprints and the aromatics upon which they are built. Using herbs and spices will up your game and keep kitchen boredom at bay. This I guarantee.

GLOBAL FLAVORPRINTS

REGION	INGREDIENT
Asian	cardamom, chiles, cilantro, cinnamon, cloves, coriander, cumin, curry powder, garlic, ginger, mint, mustard seeds, nutmeg, red pepper flakes, saffron, sesame seeds, turmeric
Mediterranean	basil, bay leaves, fennel, garlic, marjoram, mint, nutmeg, oregano, parsley, red pepper flakes, rosemary, saffron, sage, thyme
Middle Eastern	allspice, cilantro, cinnamon, coriander, cumin, garlic, marjoram, mint, oregano, sesame seeds, thyme
Moroccan	cilantro, cinnamon, coriander, cumin, garlic, ginger, mint, red pepper flakes, saffron, thyme, turmeric

Developing Your Culinary Mind

They say in life that you shouldn't sweat the small stuff. So it goes in the kitchen. Many people are amazed to find that stepping into the kitchen is actually a relaxing, almost meditative experience. There's a flow that takes place, an engagement of the mind that leaves us feeling refreshed and connected, as though all our senses were taken on a adventurous sojourn. Food and cooking demand that you be in the present, a place where yesterday's follies and tomorrow's peccadillos hold no sway. But to be fully present, it helps to learn a few tricks of the trade as a way of turning your kitchen into an inviting space filled with culinary gifts that feed the soul.

A lot of the art of developing your culinary mind comes down to time management. First, that means committing the time to get the job done. Fortunately, once you get past the learning curve, far less time is involved than you might imagine. You might well find you even have more time on your hands than you would if you were schlepping out to restaurants for meals.

There are four basic elements of time you need to budget for, and they often don't happen concurrently: planning time, shopping time, prep time, and cooking time. (There's also clean up time, but unless you're living alone, that's time I always delegate to someone else. If they're going to enjoy the fruits of my labor, they can wash a few dishes and pots.)

Just ask TV or film producers, and they'll tell you that every minute spent on planning time (aka preproduction time) saves ten minutes when the cameras finally begin to roll. Similarly, you'll save lot of time in the kitchen if you plan your meals beforehand. So, where to start?

I suggest browsing through the recipes in this book to get an idea of what strikes your fancy. Make a list of the ingredients. At first, you may have to shop for all of them, but quite quickly you'll find that you'll have many of the staples (notably the herbs and spices) in your pantry, cutting down on shopping time.

Regarding shopping time, yes, once in a while you'll find yourself doing a major shop. But more often, especially if you know which recipes you want to prepare, you'll find a quick fifteen-minute trip sometime during the day will suffice—just enough time to pick up a fresh piece of meat or some vegetables.

Prep time is where you'll save the most time and most of your sanity. There's nothing worse than coming home hungry and looking into the fridge only to see a forest of uncut veggies. That'll make you slam the door shut and reach for the phone to call the nearest Chinese restaurant for delivery. No, the right time to prep, especially vegetables, is as soon you get them home. A quick trim works wonders for taming veggies into workable components that are ready to cook—and that take up far less space in the fridge.

Everything you prep in advance is like a deposit in the culinary bank. There's nothing better—or more stress-relieving—than knowing you've got most of the components for a meal all ready to go. The whole idea is that making a meal shouldn't feel like a competition where you're rushed to get shopping, prepping, and cooking done in an impossibly short amount of time (in other words it shouldn't feel like *Top Chef*, where you're afraid the gong is going to go off halfway through your work). Cooking, the *best* cooking, almost invariably results from being relaxed rather than rushed.

Make It Ahead Strategies

I love passing along tricks of the trade. Think of this section as the Cliff Notes version of getting the most out of your prep time, and in turn, maximizing the number of recipes you'll try in the book. I think you'll be pleasantly surprised at the numerous ways you can save time with ingredients by planning ahead. Now go to it!

SPICE BLENDS. Having spice blends already mixed saves time. Make small batches to keep them fresh, and store them in little jars. Some blends essential to recipes in this book include the Classic Magic Mineral Broth combination of kombu, bay leaf, allspice berries, and peppercorns (see page 44) and *za'atar*, the versatile Middle Eastern spice blend that is typically used to season meats, vegetables, hummus, or yogurt (see page 119).

A combination of crushed or ground cumin and coriander is essential for either Toasty Spiced Roasted Potatoes (page 101) or Toasty Spiced Pumpkin Seeds (page 159); you can even use it for Kale Quinoa Salad with Red Grapes (page 89). The spice blends in Apple Pie–Spiced Walnuts and Raisins (page 161), Rosemary and Pear Muffins (page 153), and Triple Triple Brittle (page 156) can all be used interchangeably.

TOASTED NUTS AND NUT BLENDS. Toasting nuts and seeds in advance will save you a step when preparing Watercress, Purple Cabbage, and Edamame Salad with Toasted Sesame Seeds (page 75), Technicolor Slaw (page 73), Orange Salad with Olives and Mint (page 81), Kale with Delicata Squash and Hazelnuts (page 84), Roasted Orange Sesame Carrots (page 93), or Shrimp Stuffed Avocados 2.0 (page 104). The nut-and-spice blends for Tart Cherry and Chocolate Crunch (page 149) and Triple Triple Brittle (page 156) can be made in advance: toss all the dry ingredients in a bag and put in the freezer. Then, when you want one of these anytime foods, just add the wet ingredients to the nut-spice blend and pop in the oven—it's a cinch!

STOCKS. When you're home for the day, why not set a pot of Classic Magic Mineral Broth (page 44) or Old-Fashioned Chicken Stock (page 46) on the stove to do the work while you do other things? Freeze it in quart containers, so you can whip up a nourishing soup at a moments notice.

DOLLOPS. Dollops are vinaigrettes, salsas, sauces—chapter 8 has seventeen of these versatile flavor boosters. Make one or two each week to add to salads, roasted vegetables, avocado, eggs, fish, seafood, or chicken.

GREENS. To prep greens, from spinach to kale to lettuce, wash the leaves and dry them as well as possible, then as appropriate, strip them from their tough stems and tear and chop the leaves into manageable pieces. Store prepared greens in a plastic bag with a paper towel to absorb any excess water; poke a few holes in the bag to let them breathe. You can toss these ready-to-go greens into soups or salads or use them as a bed for anything warm.

FRESH VEGETABLES. After bringing vegetables home from the market, wash, dry, and chop them, then store them in the refrigerator. When you're ready to make a recipe, you can pull them out, just as you would a spice jar. Blanching and shocking broccoli (partially cooking in boiling salted water for 30 seconds and plunging into cold water to stop the cooking process) in advance will get it ready to toss onto a sheet pan to roast or into a sauté pan to finish in a few minutes.

ROASTED VEGETABLES. Some roasted vegetables banked in the refrigerator can be quickly turned into a great snack or meal. Roasted sweet potatoes, for example, can be whipped up into Curry Spiced Sweet Potato Hummus (page 148) or Sweet Potato Hash (page 135), or added to the Cozy Lentil Soup with Delicata Squash (page 59) in place of the squash, or tossed into kale or a salad. The sky's the limit.

COOKIE DOUGH. Sometimes all you want is one little sweet bite—and a whole batch of freshly baked cookies would be too tempting. So make the dough, drop it by spoonfuls onto a parchment-lined baking sheet, and freeze for an hour. Then transfer the dough balls to an airtight container or ziplock bag. Whenever you need a fix, you can pop one or two in the oven.

EXTRA INGREDIENTS. If a recipe calls for a medium onion and you only have a large one, cut the whole thing and save some in the fridge. It's great to have chopped onions, minced garlic, shredded greens, and so on ready to go and waiting for you.

Culinary Choreography

The best way to choreograph cooking time is to work from the outside in, the outside being whatever will take the longest time to cook or can be made in advance, down to those items that only need a few minutes of stove time or need to be served immediately. If you want a visual for this process, think of those Russian matryoshka dolls that nest one inside another.

I'll use Roasted Ginger Salmon with Pomegranate Olive Mint Salsa (page 114) and Ginger Scented Forbidden Rice (page 143) as an example. Here, the salmon takes the longest time to prepare and cook: it spends 20 minutes marinating and 15 minutes in the oven. But here's how to ensure you don't have wasted time. While the salmon marinates, you prep your rice (5 minutes) and get it on the stove, and, while you're there, turn on the oven to preheat for the salmon. Once the rice is on the stove (30 minutes), you turn your attention to prepping the pomegranate olive mint salsa, which takes around 10 minutes. So here's the picture so far; the salmon is marinating, the rice is cooking, the salsa is being made. When you finish the salsa, it's pretty much time to move the salmon to the oven. Once done, this leaves you 10 minutes or so to pull together a salad. If the dance is done just right, the salmon, rice, and salad will all finish around the same time, with the dollop of salsa all ready to go.

And that's for feeding four to six people!

If you're wondering how you're going to memorize all these dance moves, my response is, "don't bother." Seriously. Eventually, the timing will come naturally, but every cook I know uses a series of timers at first (and many never lose the habit). Especially if you live in a house full of distractions, timers can be your best friends, keeping you on track no matter what the interruption.

Kitchen Clarity

Your mom used to say "a place for everything, and everything in its place." Well, at least *my* mom did. That's a good rule of thumb to apply to the kitchen. Organizing a kitchen is an absolute must if you really want to enjoy cooking. Believe me, I know . . . kitchens attract stuff. All kinds of stuff, some of which has nothing to do with cooking (newspapers, mail, coloring books, keys, sunglasses, flotsam, jetsam, the works). Then there's the stuff that actually belongs in the kitchen, but like wayward bunnies, somehow manages to multiply and take over your drawers. Not long ago I did an overhaul of my own kitchen and pulled *everything* out of the drawers and cabinets. I nearly burst into tears. No wonder there was clutter. Did I really need a *dozen* vegetable peelers? Or three cherry pitters? No, I didn't, and neither do you. Here's what you do need within arm's reach of the stove:

- 1 pair of tongs
- 1 Microplane
- 1 wooden spoon
- 1 spatula
- 1 large knife
- 1 set of measuring cups
- 1 set of measuring spoons

There, that has a shot at staying pretty neat and tidy, doesn't it?

Another thing to organize is your herbs and spices. Put it this way; if those ingredients are waaaaaay back in a dark cabinet, you simply won't use them, which will be a huge disappointment to both your taste buds and your brain (brains love herbs and spices). If you're fortunate, you'll have a pullout spice rack or one that can live on the wall or counter near the stove. Failing that, put your herbs and spices at the front of a cabinet. That way, they'll always be ready to use on a moment's notice.

A lot of people think they need a large space to cook efficiently. I disagree. I've done hundreds of demos on the road, and all I usually have is two folding tables, a power strip, and a garbage pail. The key for me is in knowing where everything is before I start—pots, pans, utensils, cooking oils, seasonings, oven mitts: the lot. If you want to achieve kitchen clarity, make sure everything you use regularly has a dedicated spot, and stick to it. After a while you won't even be thinking twice about what's where; it'll always be there when you reach for it.

Reducing Recipe Reading Anxiety

Many cooks, myself included, work intuitively, adding a pinch of this, a dash of that . . . . Being intuitive is all good and fine, and quite useful when it comes to creating a recipe, but as for *re-creating* it—as in, writing it down—well, Houston, we have a problem. I used to cringe when, after I made a meal for people, they would ask the dreaded question: "Do you have a recipe for this?"

I would politely scrawl some hieroglyphics on a napkin, hoping that would appease the interested party. Then, more than a dozen years ago, I was handed my first cookbook project, and out of necessity, I *had* to learn how to write a reproducible recipe. It was critical that these culinary blueprints set the stage for consistent outcomes and success in the kitchen. In order to embrace this new language of recipe writing, I had to understand the formula. It all starts with the ingredient list.

This is the part where, if you're like me, you may get a little anxious. One, two, three, six, ten—YIKES!!! *How* many ingredients? Once upon a time, I would glance at an ingredient list, get that glazed look in my eyes, and want to run out of the kitchen. Not a viable option for a cook. So I developed a system—at first for myself, and now for you—for breaking down a recipe so you won't feel anxious when you cook your way through this book.

First, as I've mentioned, I recommend that you skim the book and see what recipes seem appealing. As you do, you'll find a common theme. There are certain herbs and spices and pantry ingredients that weave a thread throughout the recipes. Next, stock your pantry so you have some of these ingredients on hand, that way you're three-quarters of the way to having everything you need to create some yummy dishes.

Below are the ingredients for Cozy Lentil Soup with Delicata Squash (found on page 59) to illustrate my point. The ingredient list looks long; however, close to half of the list is comprised of spices (shaded in red) and three other ingredients (in blue)—olive oil, vegetable stock, and lentils—that could easily be in your pantry and/or freezer. Once you have the pantry items separated out, you can see the other ingredients are basic vegetables (shaded in green), including onions, carrots, and celery, which can live in your refrigerator already chopped and ready to go. Kale and delicata squash may well be the only ingredients you'll need to nip in to the market for.

Sea salt	2 tablespoons extra-virgin olive oil
1 teaspoon curry powder	8 cups Classic Magic Mineral Broth (page 44) or store-bought organic vegetable broth
1/2 teaspoon ground cumin	1 cup dried green lentils, rinsed well
1/2 teaspoon ground turmeric	1 yellow onion, diced small
1/4 teaspoon ground coriander	2 carrots, peeled and diced small
1/4 teaspoon ground cinnamon	2 celery stalks, diced small
Pinch of red pepper flakes	1 medium delicata squash, peeled, seeded, and cut into 1/2-inch cubes
	1 cup tightly packed, stemmed, and thinly sliced kale

Followed as written, the recipe will yield delicious results. And it is also—like so many of the recipes in this book—both forgiving and flexible, and you can look to the variation and cook's note for ingredients to swap out, or to find helpful tips and suggestions. If you don't have a specific ingredient, that doesn't mean you can't make the recipe. No kale? How about arugula, spinach, chard, or skipping it all together? The same with the herbs and spices. If you don't have cumin, turmeric, or coriander, just add another teaspoon of curry powder.

With growing kitchen confidence and skill, you can let the recipes be a blueprint where your own culinary creativity can thrive. As you get more experienced, look for foods that have similar tastes and textures; this will expand your ability to successfully substitute and come up with recipes of your own. You'll even be able to write them down, sans hieroglyphics.

Eating Organically

As a cook, I'm often asked about the importance of eating organically. The answer has three parts. The first deals with taste: organically raised foods, to my taste buds, always have more flavor, and it's especially notable with animal proteins. If you've never had grass-fed beef or pasture-raised organic eggs—oh, my, are you in for a treat.

Second, and this is where we get into the brain health part of the equation, organically raised foods are consistently more nutrient dense, and often have more favorable nutrient profiles, than nonorganic foods.

Third, and also related to brain health, there's the question of what pesticides do to the brain. Unfortunately, research on the subject is scarce. However, enough has been uncovered to put pesticides in the "when in doubt, leave it out" category. For example, certain pesticides have been associated with Parkinson's disease, and the European Food Safety Authority announced that two types of pesticides might "affect the developing human nervous system."

Fortunately—and this is where I give a hearty cheer—organics are more plentiful (and less costly) than ever before. As their popularity has soared, organics are making their way on to more and more supermarket shelves. Of course, there's always the farmers' market, which is my favorite place to seek out foods that are grown ethically and sustainably.

You may, from time to time, find yourself in a position where you have to purchase conventionally raised produce. Though the list is a bit of a moving target, there are foods whose cultivation generally uses minimal pesticides and/or leaves a minimal pesticide residue, and there are foods that bring a heavier chemical load to the table, and should be avoided. The easiest way to keep track of which is which is to access the website of the Environmental Working Group, which put out lists such as "the dirty dozen" (avoid!) and "the clean fifteen" (eat up!) at www.ewg.org/foodnews/list.

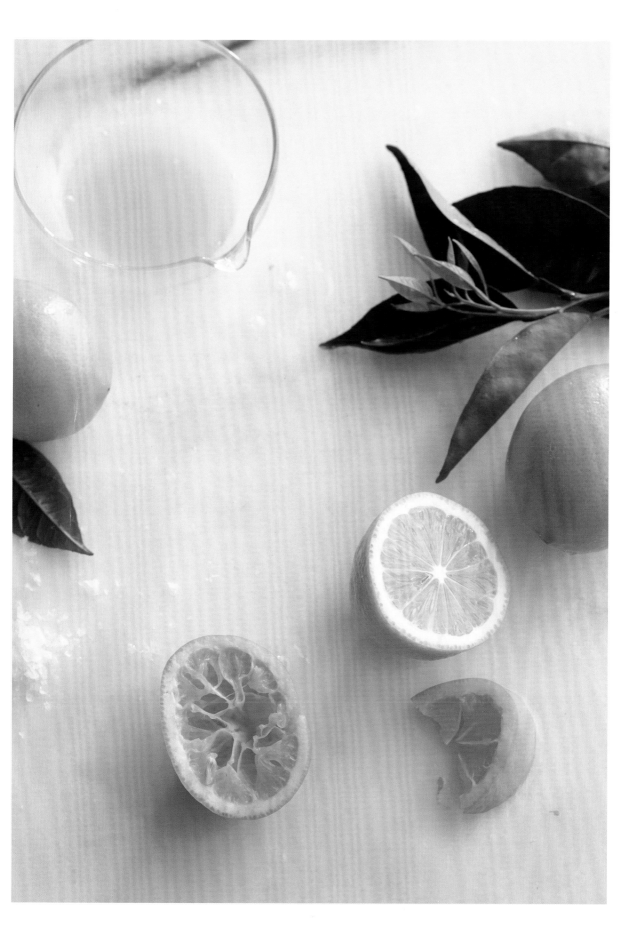

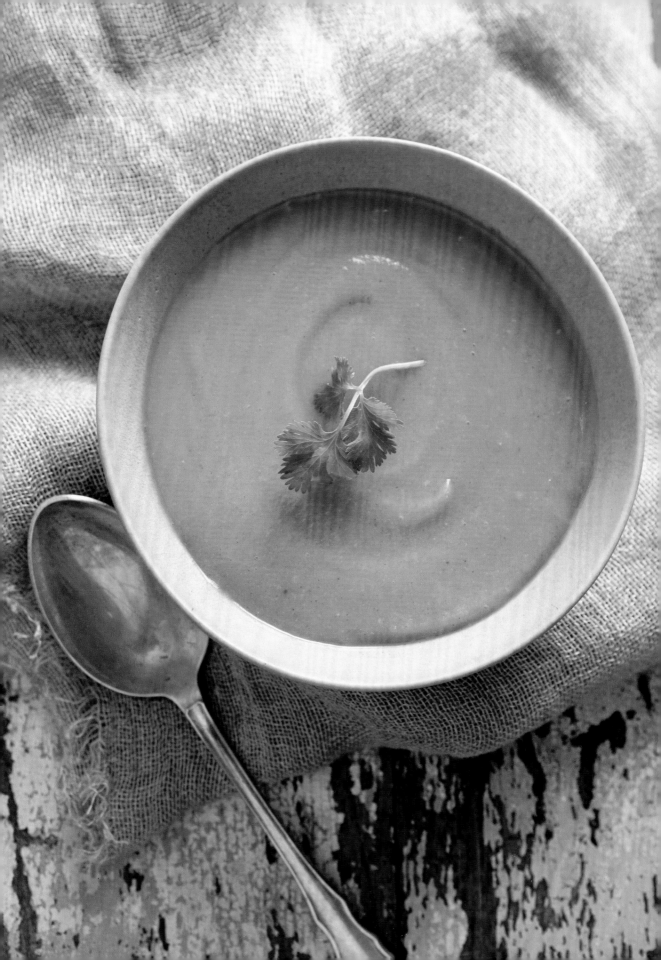

CHAPTER 4

Soups

There's no better foundation for good eating than soups. Think about it: people who wouldn't go near some lonely lentils or forlorn kale sitting alone on a plate will embrace them whole-heartedly in soups. Why is this so? It's a combination of taste, texture, and what I call the "culinary hug" provided by a warm bowl of comfort. Let's break it down. Consider the starting point for the soups in this book. The stocks in these sixteen recipes aren't water, but rather my signature Classic Magic Mineral Broth (page 44) or Old-Fashioned Chicken Stock (page 46). These soup bases are incredibly nutrient dense, with loads of brain-healthy minerals such as phosphorus, magnesium, and potassium. And, from a texture viewpoint, the vegetable's fibers have been broken down, making them easy to chew and digest while still retaining all their earthy tastes. Those tastes can be perfectly balanced using a great, simple tool called FASS (see page 30). Even if I didn't add a single ingredient to the base stock, the heady flavors would be enough to put a smile on your face and some serious heat in your belly. But I'm never satisfied with "just enough" taste. I want more, more, more!!!—and soup is the perfect delivery vehicle. It's incredibly versatile, meaning I can choose a flavorprint—Moroccan, Middle Eastern, Italian, pick a region—and easily work those vegetables, herbs, and spices (many of which have brain-protecting properties) into the pot. There I watch the magic of culinary alchemy take place, as the liquid and heat break down what might otherwise be challenging ingredients, transforming them into something delicious. I'm a soup person at heart, in part because it's so much fun to teach people how to make them, course-correct them, and enjoy them by the mug, cup, or bowl. If any group of recipes can satisfy body and soul, and boost your mood in the process, it's these soups.

Classic Magic Mineral Broth

MAKES ABOUT 6 QUARTS • PREP TIME: 10 minutes • COOK TIME: 2 to 4 hours

All cooks like to think that, at some point in their careers, they've contributed something to the greater culinary canon. Well, this broth is my signature, and I'm amazed and humbled at the reaction it's garnered over the years. It's sort of like a pebble tossed into a lake; you can't imagine how far the ripples will reach. I knew, from a taste perspective, that it was versatile, delicious, and nutrient dense; indeed, it's the base for most of my soups. But as research has progressed over the past decade, it's uncanny how incredibly healthy this soup has turned out to be for all parts of the body, including the brain. It's loaded with magnesium, which is incredibly calming. And science has even explained its popularity—the sweet potatoes and kombu provide a sense of umami, a savory taste that scientists claim is the hidden element behind cravings. If you're going to have cravings, this is one of the healthiest and tastiest you can indulge. Some people call it the magic broth, others call it the miracle broth; I just call it a culinary touchstone for everything good that food can bring to your mind and body.

6 unpeeled carrots, rinsed well and cut in thirds

2 unpeeled yellow onions, rinsed well and cut into chunks

1 leek, white and green parts, rinsed well and cut in thirds

1 bunch celery, including the heart, rinsed well and cut in thirds

4 unpeeled red potatoes, rinsed well and quartered

2 unpeeled Japanese or regular sweet potatoes, rinsed well and quartered

1 unpeeled Garnet yam (sweet potato), rinsed well and quartered

5 unpeeled cloves garlic, rinsed well and halved

1/2 bunch fresh flat-leaf parsley

1 (8-inch) strip of kombu

12 black peppercorns

4 whole allspice or juniper berries

2 bay leaves

8 quarts cold filtered water, plus more if needed

Sea salt

In a 12-quart or larger stockpot, combine the carrots, onions, leek, celery, potatoes, sweet potatoes, yam, garlic, parsley, kombu, peppercorns, allspice berries, and bay leaves. Add the water, cover, and bring to a boil.

Decrease the heat to low and simmer, partially covered, for at least 2 hours. As the broth simmers, some of the water will evaporate; add more if the vegetables begin to peek out. Simmer until the full richness of the vegetables can be tasted.

Strain the broth through a large, coarse-mesh sieve (remember to use a heat-resistant container underneath), and discard the solids. Add 1 teaspoon sea salt, or more to taste.

Let cool to room temperature before refrigerating or freezing.

COOK'S NOTES: This recipe is designed for a 12-quart or larger stockpot. If you only have an 8-quart pot, cut the recipe in half.

Soup making will be a cinch if you keep this broth on hand; store it in 1 quart containers in the freezer. It's also great for just plain sipping.

The longer you simmer this broth, the more flavor and nutrient density it will have. If you don't want to tend to it for hours on end, you can also cut the recipe in half and make it in a slow cooker.

What is kombu? It's a long, dark brown to black seaweed that's dried and folded into sheets. Kombu is a natural flavor enhancer, and it contains a full range of trace minerals including brain-boosting potassium and vitamins A and C. It keeps indefinitely when stored in a cool, dry place. Look for it in the Asian section of your grocery store, or use the Resources on page 225.

PER SERVING: Serving Size: 1 cup; Calories: 45; Total Fat: 0 g (0 g saturated, 0 g monounsaturated); Carbohydrates: 11 g; Protein: 1 g; Fiber: 2 g; Sodium: 124 mg

STORAGE: Store in an airtight container in the refrigerator for 5 to 7 days or in the freezer for 4 months.

Old-Fashioned Chicken Stock

MAKES ABOUT 6 QUARTS · PREP TIME: 10 minutes · COOK TIME: 3 hours

Maybe it's because, at heart, I'm a soup maker, but I take making stock *very* seriously. I think most cooks feel that way. There's a confidence one gets in making one's own stock rather than buying the boxed version. (Organic chicken stock will do in a pinch, but give me my own heady concoction any day.) I get to control the ingredients and, as with this chicken stock, get the taste exactly the way I want. A big plus is that it freezes well for storage. This stock, along with Classic Magic Mineral Broth (page 44), is the base for nearly every soup in this book, so it has to be spot on, and it is. Bone broths are some of the world's oldest healing foods, and with good reason; the calcium, magnesium, and phosphorus in chicken bones are great for brain health, while the amino acid glycine has calming and other mental health benefits.

6 pounds organic chicken backs, necks, bones, and wings

2 unpeeled white onions, coarsely chopped

4 unpeeled large carrots, cut in thirds

2 celery stalks, cut in thirds

6 fresh thyme sprigs

4 cloves garlic, unpeeled and smashed

1 large bunch fresh flat-leaf parsley

1 bay leaf

8 black peppercorns

8 quarts cold filtered water, plus more if needed

In a 12-quart or larger stockpot, combine the chicken, onions, carrots, celery, thyme, garlic, parsley, bay leaf, and peppercorns. Add the water, cover, and heat over medium-high heat until the water comes to a boil. Lower the heat so the bubbles just break the surface of the liquid. Skim off the scum and the fat that has risen to the surface. Simmer partially covered for about 3 hours. Add more water if too much has evaporated.

Strain the stock through a fine-mesh sieve or colander lined with unbleached cheesecloth into a clean pot or heat-resistant bowl. Bring to room temperature before covering and storing in the refrigerator. The next day, spoon off and discard any fat that has risen to the surface, and refrigerate or freeze.

COOK'S NOTES: This recipe is designed for a 12-quart or larger stockpot. If you only have an 8-quart pot, cut the recipe in half.

Stock can be frozen for up to 3 months. Store stock in various sizes of containers so that you can pull out a cup for deglazing or a quart or two to make a pot of soup.

The stock will cool faster in smaller containers. Make sure it's refrigerated within 4 hours.

PER SERVING: Serving Size: 1 cup; Calories: 50; Total Fat: 1.5 g (0 g saturated, 0 g monounsaturated); Carbohydrates: 3 g; Protein: 1.2 g; Fiber: 1 g; Sodium: 144 mg

STORAGE: Store in an airtight container in the refrigerator for 5 to 7 days or in the freezer for 4 months.

Gingered Butternut Squash Soup
WITH WALNUT CREAM

MAKES 6 SERVINGS • PREP TIME: 15 minutes • COOK TIME: 20 minutes

There's something invigorating about the fall. The crispness in the air, the world settling down for a long siesta . . . these changes around me, trigger changes in the kitchen. My bellwether of the season to come is butternut squash soup. The squash is high in potassium and vitamin B6, which benefits nerve health, and paired with apple and ginger it is as soothing as it gets. The walnut cream gives the soup that satiating taste that befits the feeling of coming home after a brisk fall walk.

To make the walnut cream, combine the walnuts, water, lemon juice, maple syrup, sea salt, and nutmeg in a blender or food processor. Process until creamy smooth, about two minutes, and set aside.

To make the soup, heat the olive oil in a soup pot over medium heat, then add the onion, shallot, and a pinch of salt. Sauté until golden and translucent, about 4 minutes. Add ginger, allspice, cinnamon, and red pepper flakes and sauté 1 minute longer. Add the butternut squash, apple, and $1/2$ teaspoon of salt, stirring and cooking for another 2 to 3 minutes. Pour in $1/2$ cup of the broth to deglaze the pan, stirring to loosen any bits stuck to the pot, and cook until the liquid is reduced by half. Add the remaining $4^1/2$ cups of broth. Bring to a boil over high heat, then reduce the heat to medium low, cover, and simmer until the squash is tender, about 15 minutes.

In a blender, puree the soup in batches until very smooth, adding more broth or water if you'd like a thinner soup. Return the soup to the pot and gently reheat. Taste; you may want to add a pinch of salt, a drop of maple syrup, or a squeeze of lemon juice. Serve garnished with 1 teaspoon of walnut cream in each bowl. Store the walnut cream in an airtight container and keep in the refrigerator for up to five days or the freezer for later use.

COOK'S NOTE: If you don't want to take out your chainsaw, many grocers have done the heavy lifting for you. Look for precut butternut squash cubes in the produce section. For this recipe, you'll need about 5 cups.

PER SERVING: Calories: 139; Total Fat: 5 g (1 g saturated, 4 g mono-unsaturated); Carbohydrates: 25 g; Protein: 2 g; Fiber: 5 g; Sodium: 160 mg

STORAGE: Store in an airtight container in the refrigerator for up to 5 days or in the freezer for up to 2 months.

WALNUT CREAM

1 cup walnuts, toasted

$3/4$ cup water

2 teaspoons freshly squeezed lemon juice

$1/4$ teaspoon sea salt

$1/4$ teaspoon Grade B maple syrup

Fresh grating of nutmeg

SOUP

2 tablespoons extra-virgin olive oil

1 small yellow onion, diced

1 small shallot, chopped

Sea salt

1 tablespoon minced fresh ginger

$1/4$ teaspoon ground allspice

$1/2$ teaspoon ground cinnamon

$1/4$ teaspoon red pepper flakes

$1^1/2$ pounds butternut squash, peeled and cut into 1-inch cubes

1 Granny Smith apple, peeled, cored, and chopped

5 cups Classic Magic Mineral Broth (page 44) or store-bought organic vegetable broth, plus more if needed

Grade B maple syrup

Freshly squeezed lemon juice

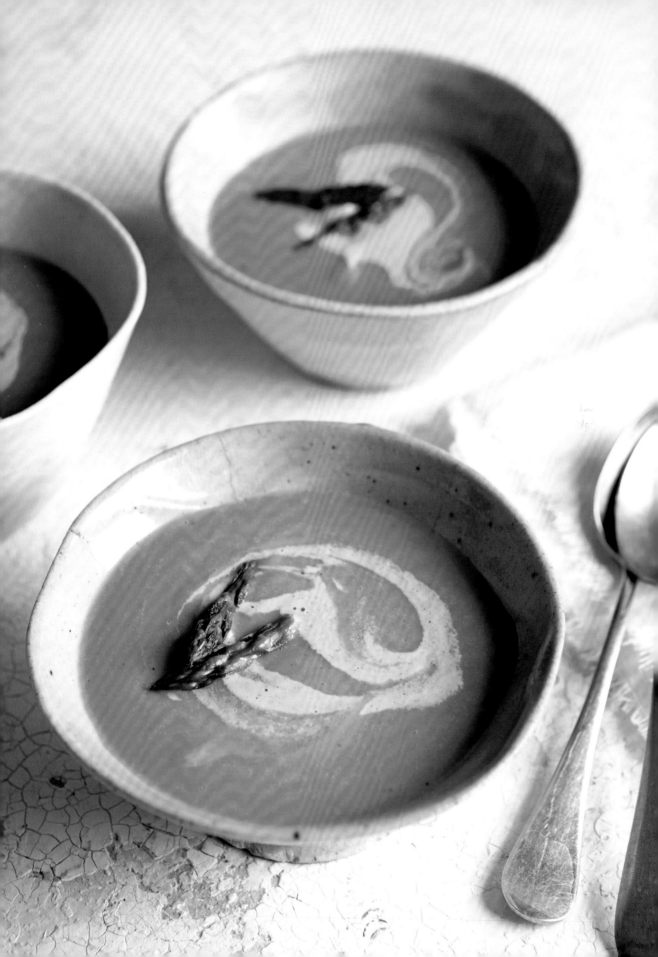

Roasted Asparagus Soup
WITH PISTACHIO CREAM

MAKES 6 SERVINGS · PREP TIME: 10 minutes · COOK TIME: 20 minutes

Gone are the days when asparagus was boiled until it resembled a gray Seattle drizzle. Here we roast asparagus until it becomes sweet and caramelized in a way that's hard to believe until it's tried. Asparagus is full of antioxidants that help in DNA synthesis and repair. In this soup, it's paired with the nerve-protective benefits of pistachio as part of the minty, creamy topping. This is some serious yum in a bowl.

Preheat the oven to 400°F.

To make the pistachio cream, put the water, pistachios, mint, lemon juice, and 1/4 teaspoon of salt in a blender or food processor and process until smooth and creamy. Taste; you may want to add a bit more salt.

Cut off the asparagus tips and put the stalks and tips on a rimmed baking sheet in a single layer. Drizzle the asparagus with 1 tablespoon of the olive oil and sprinkle with 1/4 teaspoon of salt. Toss evenly to coat. Bake for 8 to 10 minutes, until tender. Remove the asparagus tips from the baking sheet and reserve for garnishing the soup.

Heat the remaining 2 tablespoons of olive oil in an 8-quart pot over medium heat. Add the onion, leeks, and a pinch of salt. Sauté for 4 minutes, then add the potato and a generous pinch of salt. Stir occasionally, allowing the potatoes to soften and the onion to turn golden. Add the garlic and sauté for 30 seconds. Pour in 1 cup of the broth and deglaze the pot, stirring to loosen any bits stuck to the pot. Add the remaining 5 cups of broth and bring to a boil. Decrease the heat to low and simmer for 5 minutes.

In batches, puree the soup in a blender, adding the broth first, then the vegetables and asparagus. Blend until velvety smooth, about 2 minutes. If the soup is too thick, add more broth 1/2 cup at a time. Return the soup to the pot and gently reheat. Taste; you may want to add a pinch of salt or a squeeze of lemon.

Stir 1 cup of the pistachio cream into the soup. Ladle the soup into bowls and garnish with the reserved asparagus tips.

CONTINUED

PISTACHIO CREAM

1 cup water or organic broth or stock

1 cup shelled pistachios

1 tablespoon chopped mint

2 teaspoons freshly squeezed lemon juice

Sea salt

SOUP

2 bunches of asparagus (about 2 pounds), tough ends snapped off, remaining stalks peeled

3 tablespoons extra-virgin olive oil

Sea salt

1 small yellow onion, diced

2 leeks, white part only, chopped

1 Yellow Finn or Yukon gold potato, peeled and diced

2 cloves garlic, chopped

6 cups Classic Magic Mineral Broth (page 44), Old-Fashioned Chicken Stock (page 46), or store-bought organic stock, plus more if needed

Roasted Asparagus Soup, *continued*

COOK'S NOTES: For an ultrasmooth velvety texture, go one step further: strain through a fine-mesh sieve, using the back of a wooden spoon to push the liquid through.

The ends of the asparagus can be stringy, so peeling just the ends will ensure that you have the smoothest soup possible.

PER SERVING: Calories: 300; Total Fat: 15 g (2 g saturated, 9.5 g mono-unsaturated); Carbohydrates: 30 g; Protein: 10 g; Fiber: 9 g; Sodium: 433 mg

STORAGE: Store in an airtight container in the refrigerator for up to 5 days or in the freezer for up to 1 month.

Curried Zucchini Soup

MAKES 8 SERVINGS · PREP TIME: 10 minutes · COOK TIME: 25 minutes

Zucchinis are like the rabbits of the vegetable kingdom; they tend to grow and multiply prolifically. I found that out the first summer I grew them out here in California. One morning I had a few tiny, cute zucchini buds in the garden; the next day, *whammo!,* I had a whole family of the critters. I wish I'd had a time-lapse camera documenting the process, as it really did seem to happen that quickly. Given the plethora of zucchini around here come July and August, you need to get creative to stay one step ahead of the game. I find zucchini pairs wonderfully with yogurt (which has great probiotics) and with the rich wonders of anti-inflammatory turmeric. As with all my cold soups, I like to serve these as shooters in little glasses. No spoon required.

Heat the olive oil in a sauté pan over medium heat, then add the onion and a pinch of salt and sauté until golden, about 5 minutes. Add the garlic, curry powder, cumin, potato, and another pinch of salt. Continue to sauté for a minute. Pour in $1/2$ cup of the broth to deglaze the pan, stirring to loosen any bits stuck to the pan, and cook until the liquid is reduced by half and the potatoes begin to get tender, about 1 to 2 minutes. Add 1 tablespoon of broth if they begin to stick or the pan gets too dry. Add the zucchini, $1/4$ teaspoon of salt, and the black pepper. Stir to coat and sauté for a few minutes. Pour in the remaining broth. Cover and cook over medium heat for 10 minutes or until the zucchini is tender.

Ladle the soup into the blender in batches, adding the liquid first, then the solids. Blend until very smooth, about 2 minutes. Add lemon juice and salt to taste.

Chill the soup for 2 hours, then whisk in the yogurt. Taste; you may want to add a pinch of salt or a squeeze of lemon juice. Serve in bowls or small glasses garnished with the mint and parsley.

COOK'S NOTE: If you just can't wait until it's chilled, eat this soup hot, warm, or at room temperature.

PER SERVING: Calories: 173; Total Fat: 9 g (4 g saturated, 4 g mono-unsaturated); Carbohydrates: 19 g; Protein: 5.5 g; Fiber: 4 g; Sodium: 219 mg

STORAGE: Store in an airtight container in the refrigerator for up to 5 days or in the freezer for up to 1 month.

2 tablespoons extra-virgin olive oil

1 yellow onion, finely diced

Sea salt

2 cloves garlic, minced

1 tablespoon curry powder

1 teaspoon ground cumin

1 red potato, peeled and diced small

4 cups Classic Magic Mineral Broth (page 44) or store-bought organic vegetable broth

$1 1/2$ pounds zucchini, quartered lengthwise, then cut crosswise into $1/2$-inch pieces

$1/8$ teaspoon freshly ground pepper

Freshly squeezed lemon juice

1 cup organic plain Greek yogurt

1 tablespoon chopped fresh mint, for garnish

2 tablespoons chopped cilantro, for garnish

Clean Green Soup

MAKES 6 SERVINGS · PREP TIME: 15 minutes · COOK TIME: 20 minutes

Here's a recipe where, if it's leafy and green, it'll work. I use chard and collards, but kale or spinach would be brilliant too—in fact, put it this way: if you think Popeye would eat it, it's in. The flavor enhancers are onion, garlic, red pepper flakes, and lemon zest, with a yellow potato thrown in for creaminess. The whole pot gets blended, and you'll swear you're eating emeralds (albeit luscious ones): that's how shimmering green this soup looks. It's a smart, calming soup, with whichever cruciferous greens you use (kale, bok choy, watercress, collards) providing a ton of folate, which may help ward off depression.

Extra-virgin olive oil

1 large yellow onion, diced

1 large Yukon gold or Yellow Finn potato, peeled and diced small

Sea salt

2 teaspoons minced garlic

1 generous pinch red pepper flakes

6 cups Classic Magic Mineral Broth (page 44) or store-bought organic vegetable broth, plus an extra cup if needed

1 bunch collards, stemmed and coarsely chopped

1 bunch green chard, stemmed and coarsely chopped

1 cup loosely packed chopped fresh parsley

1 teaspoon lemon zest

1 tablespoon freshly squeezed lemon juice

Heat 2 tablespoons of the olive oil in a soup pot over medium heat, then add the onion, potato, and $1/4$ teaspoon of salt and sauté until the onion is golden, about 10 minutes. Add the garlic and red pepper flakes and stir for another 30 seconds. Pour in $1/2$ cup of the broth, stirring to loosen any bits stuck to the pot, and cook until the liquid is reduced by half.

Add in the collards and chard and another $1/4$ teaspoon of salt. Stir well to combine so that the greens will wilt. Then add the remaining $5^1/2$ cups of broth, bring to a boil, reduce the heat to medium, cover, and simmer for 5 minutes.

In a blender, puree the soup in batches until very smooth, each time adding the cooking liquid first and then the greens mixture. Blend the parsley into the last batch. Pour the soup back into the pot, heat gently, and stir in the lemon zest and juice. Taste; you may want to add a pinch more salt. Serve garnished with a drizzle of olive oil.

COOK'S NOTE: Here's an important physics-based safety note: blending hot liquids causes pressure to rise in the blender jar, which can blow the lid right off. To help prevent this, leave at least one-third of the jar empty. Another way to be safe, avoiding both burns and unwanted spin art on your kitchen walls, is to seal the blender lid tightly, put a kitchen towel over the lid, and hold the lid in place before you hit the power button. And always add liquid to the jar first, then solids, for the smoothest blending.

PER SERVING: Calories: 145; Total Fat: 5 g (1 g saturated, 4 g mono-unsaturated); Carbohydrates: 22 g; Protein: 4 g; Fiber: 6 g; Sodium: 439 mg

STORAGE: Store in an airtight container in the refrigerator for up to 5 days or in the freezer for up to 1 month.

Summer's Best Roasted Tomato
AND RED BELL PEPPER SOUP

MAKES 4 SERVINGS · PREP TIME: 15 minutes · COOK TIME: 30 minutes

I'm a big believer in seasonal cooking. You get the best taste, because you're eating foods at their peak, and it's also cheaper than buying the same foods that are trucked/shipped/space-shuttled in off-season from who knows where. Heirloom tomatoes and red peppers tend to appear simultaneously at the farmers' market in the summertime, and both are a veritable lycopene fest. Lycopene is a super antioxidant that fights inflammation and, potentially, depression. You'll definitely be uplifted eating this soup, which is topped with a basil cashew cream.

Preheat the oven to 400°F.

In a bowl, combine the tomatoes, bell pepper, onion, garlic, thyme, oregano, olive oil, 1/2 teaspoon of salt, and pepper and mix to evenly coat. Spread the vegetables evenly on a parchment-lined baking sheet. Roast for 30 minutes, turning the baking sheet halfway through, until the vegetables are lightly golden and soft.

Pick up the parchment paper by the corners and pour the vegetables, plus any liquid, into your blender. Add the broth and blend on high for at least 1 minute, until smooth and creamy. Add the basil and give a few pulses, until the basil is combined. Taste; you may want to add a pinch or two of salt, a splash of lemon juice, or a drop or two of maple syrup.

The soup can be served at room temperature, gently heated, or chilled. Before serving, add a tablespoon of the basil cashew cream to each serving.

PER SERVING: Calories: 147; Total Fat: 8 g (1g saturated, 5.5 g mono-unsaturated); Carbohydrates: 18.5 g; Protein: 3.5 g; Fiber: 5.5 g; Sodium: 338 mg

STORAGE: Store in an airtight container in the refrigerator for up to 5 days or in the freezer for up to 2 months.

2 pounds heirloom tomatoes, quartered

1 large red bell pepper, seeded, stemmed, and cut in six pieces

1 small red onion, cut in large chunks

2 cloves garlic, peeled

1 tablespoon minced fresh thyme

1 tablespoon minced fresh oregano

2 tablespoons extra-virgin olive oil

Sea salt

1/4 teaspoon freshly ground black pepper

3 cups Classic Magic Mineral Broth (page 44) or store-bought organic vegetable broth, at room temperature

1 cup loosely packed basil leaves

Freshly squeezed lemon juice

Grade B maple syrup

6 tablespoons Basil Cashew Cream (page 179)

Moroccan Chickpea and Vegetable Soup

MAKES 6 SERVINGS • PREP TIME: 15 minutes • COOK TIME: 25 minutes

I knew I was on the right track with this soup when Catherine, my scrupulous recipe tester for the past seven years, wrote the following reaction to trying it: "Nothing to say but *swooooooooon.*'" Now that's what I call positive feedback! The trick with this soup is that after I cook it, I take half of it out of the pot and blend it, and back into the pot it goes. It's an act of culinary prestidigitation: the blending will make you think there are three cartons of cream added to the soup, but 'tis not the case. There are plenty of brain boosters in this soup, notably the spices; curcumin has been shown to fight depression, and may play a role in the production of brain-derived neurotrophic factors, genes that help with memory and learning and help brain neurons function and survive.

2 tablespoons extra-virgin olive oil

2 small yellow onions, diced small

1 fennel bulb, diced small

2 stalks celery, chopped

Sea salt

1 small sweet potato, peeled and cut into $1/2$-inch dice

1 carrot, peeled and diced small

1 large clove garlic, minced

1 teaspoon ground cumin

$1/2$ teaspoon ground turmeric

$1/4$ teaspoon ground coriander

$1/4$ teaspoon ground cinnamon

Pinch of red pepper flakes

Pinch of saffron (optional)

6 cups Classic Magic Mineral Broth (page 44) or store-bought organic vegetable broth

4 cups cooked chickpeas, or 2 (15-ounce cans), rinsed

Freshly squeezed lemon juice

Freshly ground black pepper

Grade B maple syrup (optional)

2 tablespoons chopped fresh cilantro, for garnish

1 tablespoon chopped fresh mint, for garnish

Heat the olive oil in a soup pot over medium heat, then add the onions, fennel, celery, and a pinch of salt and sauté until golden, about 6 minutes. Add the sweet potato and carrot and sauté another 3 minutes. Add the garlic and cook for 30 seconds. Stir in the cumin, turmeric, $1/2$ teaspoon of salt, coriander, cinnamon, red pepper flakes, and saffron and stir for another 30 seconds, or until fragrant. Pour in $1/2$ cup of the broth to deglaze the pot, stirring to loosen any bits stuck to the pot, and cook until the liquid is reduced by half.

Spritz the chickpeas with lemon juice, add a pinch of salt, and stir, then add to the pot. Add the remaining $5^1/2$ cups of broth. Bring to a boil, then reduce the heat to medium, cover, and simmer for 15 minutes.

Ladle 4 cups of the soup into a blender and process for 1 minute or until velvety smooth. Stir the blended mixture back into the soup and cook over low heat, just until heated through.

Stir in 4 teaspoons of lemon juice and a few grinds of black pepper. Taste; you may want to add a pinch of salt, a drop or so of maple syrup, or a squeeze of lemon juice.

Served garnished with the cilantro and mint.

PER SERVING: Calories: 268; Total Fat: 6 g (1 g saturated, 4 g monounsaturated); Carbohydrates: 44 g; Protein: 10 g; Fiber: 10 g; Sodium: 385 mg

STORAGE: Store in an airtight container in the refrigerator for up to 5 days or in the freezer for up to 2 months.

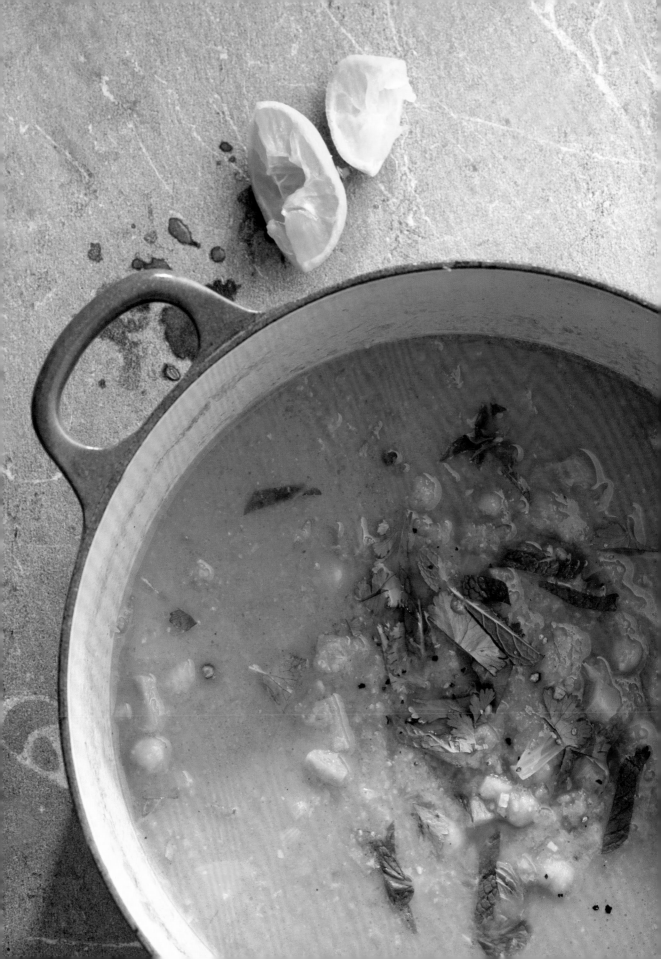

Southwestern Sweet Potato Soup

I'll admit it took a couple of takes to get this recipe to Yum! Let's just say I was little cavalier with the ancho chiles and chipotle the first time out: one taste, and I looked like a cartoon character with steam blowing out of my ears while a train whistle screams. I mean, even a dragon wouldn't have gone there, it was that hot. But a little experimentation—and pulling back on the chiles a tad—turned this former five-alarmer into an amazingly heady, slightly smoky soup. This is brain-friendly all the way; the capsaicin in chile is renowned for stimulating blood flow and releasing stress-reducing hormones, with the sweet potatoes providing a kick of beta-carotene, perhaps the most potent antioxidant.

2 tablespoons extra-virgin olive oil

1 yellow onion, diced small

Sea salt

1 red bell pepper, coarsely chopped

2 teaspoons minced garlic

2 pounds sweet potatoes, peeled and diced into 1-inch cubes

2 teaspoons ground cumin

$1/4$ teaspoon ground chipotle chile

$1/4$ teaspoon ground ancho chile

6 cups Classic Magic Mineral Broth (page 44) or store-bought organic vegetable broth, plus more as needed

1 teaspoon freshly squeezed lime juice

$1/2$ teaspoon Grade B maple syrup

1 tablespoon finely chopped cilantro, for garnish

Heat the olive oil in a soup pot over medium heat. Add the onion and a pinch of salt and sauté until translucent, about 4 minutes. Add the bell pepper, garlic, and another pinch of salt and sauté for about a minute. Add the sweet potatoes, cumin, chipotle and ancho chiles, and $1/2$ teaspoon of salt. Mix until the sweet potatoes are well coated. Add in $1/2$ cup of broth, stirring to loosen any bits stuck to the pot, and cook until the liquid is reduced by half. Add the remaining $51/2$ cups of broth and increase the heat to high; bring to a boil. Decrease the heat to medium-low to maintain a vigorous simmer until the sweet potatoes are tender, about 15 minutes.

Ladle the soup into a blender in batches and gradually bring up to high speed for about 1 minute, until the soup is smooth and creamy. If it's too thick, add more broth $1/2$ cup at a time. Pour the soup back into the pot, heat gently, stir in the lime juice and maple syrup, then taste. You may want to add another pinch or two of salt.

Garnish with the cilantro, and serve.

VARIATION: For an over-the-top garnish, add a few Toasty Spiced Pumpkin Seeds (see page 159) to each bowl.

COOK'S NOTE: Want to bring the heat? Bump up the chipotle and ancho by $1/4$ teaspoon.

PER SERVING: Calories: 210; Total Fat: 5 g (1 g saturated, 4 g mono-unsaturated); Carbohydrates: 38 g; Protein: 3 g; Fiber: 7 g; Sodium: 388 mg

STORAGE: Store in an airtight container in the refrigerator for up to 5 days or in the freezer for up to 2 months.

Not Your Grandpa's Borscht

MAKES 6 SERVINGS • PREP TIME: 15 minutes • COOK TIME: 30 minutes

Maybe it's just me, but I hear the word "borscht," and visions of Cossacks doing the Sabre Dance just pop into my head. Or maybe Billy Crystal doing shtick in the Catskills. But this isn't your great-granddaddy's old-world borscht, nor the store-bought purple miscreation foisted upon guests during the holidays. Yes, there are beets in this borscht—and a good thing, too, because beets are a fabulous brain food, as they relax the blood vessels and improve circulation. And here they look as good as they taste: diced into half-inch bites, they look like rubies in a bowl of Classic Magic Mineral Broth (page 44). Add coriander, cumin, coriander, some cabbage for depth, and caraway seeds, and you've got a concoction that would've made the Czar a convert.

Heat the olive oil in a soup pot over medium heat, then add the onion, fennel, celery, and a $^1/_2$ teaspoon of salt and sauté until golden, about 6 minutes. Stir in the cumin, coriander, caraway, and red pepper flakes and sauté until well combined. Pour in $^1/_2$ cup of the broth to deglaze the pot, stirring to loosen any bits stuck to the pot, and cook until the liquid is reduced by half.

Add the cabbage and $^1/_4$ teaspoon of salt and stir. Then add the beets and another $^1/_4$ teaspoon of salt; stir, and cook for about a minute. Add the remaining $5^1/_2$ cups of broth and another $^1/_2$ teaspoon of salt. Bring to a boil, then reduce the heat to medium, cover, and simmer until the beets are tender, about 20 to 25 minutes. Add the lemon juice and taste; you may want to add another pinch of salt or a squeeze of lemon.

Spoon the soup into bowls and garnish each with a teaspoon of yogurt and a sprinkle of dill. Serve immediately.

COOK'S NOTE: If you don't want to look like a crime suspect, you may want to wear kitchen gloves while cutting up your beets.

PER SERVING: Calories: 157; Total Fat: 8 g (1 g saturated, 6 g mono-unsaturated); Carbohydrates: 21 g; Protein: 3 g; Fiber: 6 g; Sodium: 507 mg

STORAGE: Store in an airtight container in the refrigerator for up to 5 days or in the freezer for up to 2 months.

3 tablespoons extra-virgin olive oil

1 medium onion, diced

1 fennel bulb, diced

2 celery stalks, diced

Sea salt

1 teaspoon ground cumin

1 teaspoon ground coriander

1 teaspoon caraway seeds

Pinch of red pepper flakes

6 cups Classic Magic Mineral Broth (page 44), Nourishing Bone Broth (page 67), or store-bought organic vegetable broth

3 cups $^1/_2$-inch diced green cabbage

3 beets, trimmed, peeled, and cut into $^1/_2$-inch dice

1 tablespoon freshly squeezed lemon juice

6 teaspoons plain yogurt, for garnish

$^1/_4$ cup chopped fresh dill, for garnish

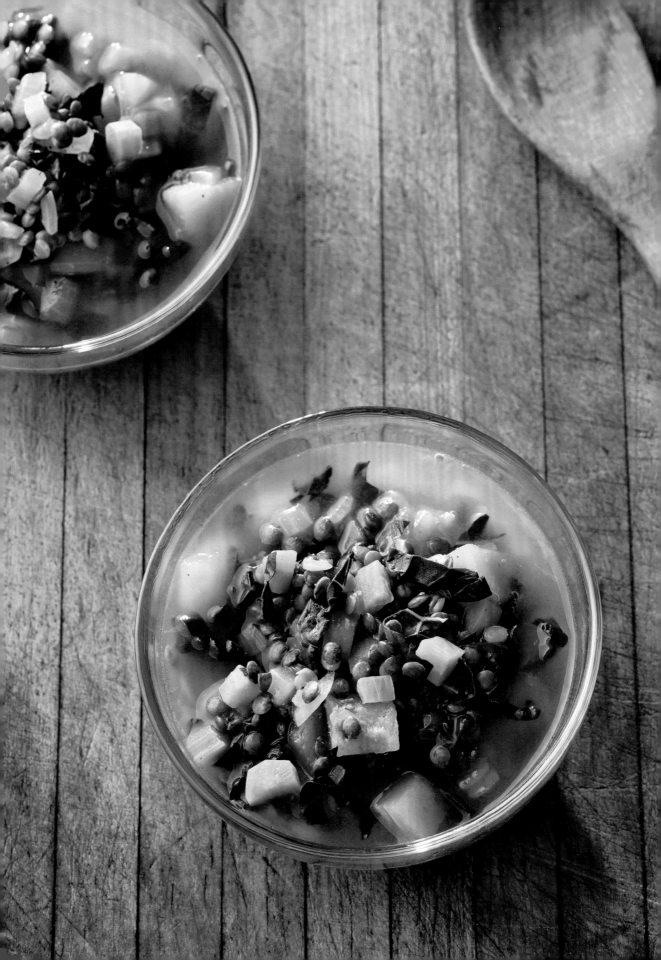

Cozy Lentil Soup
WITH DELICATA SQUASH

MAKES 6 SERVINGS · PREP TIME: 20 minutes · COOK TIME: 35 minutes

Silicon Valley has promised us that, someday, little nanobots will act like tiny microprocessors in our brains, helping to make us smarter. I say, Why wait? We already have a teensy food that does that. It's the lentil, the vegetable kingdom's version of a Lilliputian flying saucer. Lentils, ounce for ounce, pack an amazing amount of brain boosters, such as iron (essential to the function of myelin, which is involved in quick information gathering). From a culinary viewpoint, it's a myth that you have to soak lentils overnight; just a quick rinse will do. With a host of spices, cubed delicata squash, and thinly sliced kale, this is my go-to soup when I'm working hard and need to process a lot of information.

Heat the olive oil in a Dutch oven or heavy soup pot over medium heat. Add the onion and a pinch of salt and sauté until translucent, about 4 minutes. Add the carrots, celery, delicata squash, and another pinch of salt and sauté until all of the vegetables are just tender, about 5 minutes.

Add the curry powder, cumin, turmeric, coriander, cinnamon, 1/4 teaspoon of salt, and red pepper flakes and give a stir. Add the lentils and stir to coat. Pour in 1/2 cup of the broth to deglaze the pot, stirring to loosen any bits stuck to the pot, and cook until the liquid is reduced by half. Add the rest of the broth. Increase the heat to high and bring to a boil. Decrease the heat to low, cover, and simmer until the lentils are tender, about 20 to 25 minutes. Taste; you may want to add a pinch of salt. Stir in the kale and cook until it's tender, about 3 minutes.

VARIATION: Substitute fennel, which is a good digestive aid, for the celery to add more depth to the flavor.

COOK'S NOTE: If you have trouble finding delicata squash, use its cousin, butternut squash.

PER SERVING: Calories: 224; Total Fat: 6 g (1 g saturated, 4 g mono-unsaturated); Carbohydrates: 37 g; Protein: 9 g; Fiber: 10 g; Sodium: 329 mg

STORAGE: Store in an airtight container in the refrigerator for up to 5 days or in the freezer for up to 2 months.

2 tablespoons extra-virgin olive oil

1 yellow onion, diced small

Sea salt

2 carrots, peeled and diced small

2 celery stalks, diced small

1 medium delicata squash, peeled, seeded, and cut into 1/2-inch cubes

1 teaspoon curry powder

1/2 teaspoon ground cumin

1/2 teaspoon ground turmeric

1/4 teaspoon ground coriander

1/4 teaspoon ground cinnamon

Pinch of red pepper flakes

1 cup dried green lentils, rinsed well

8 cups Classic Magic Mineral Broth (page 44) or store-bought organic vegetable broth

1 cup tightly packed, stemmed, and thinly sliced kale

Sicilian Chicken Soup

This might seem like heresy coming from a nice Jewish girl such as myself, but there's more than one way to make chicken soup. Sure, there's what my nana would call "Jewish penicillin," but that kind of chicken soup tends to be bland. This Italian chicken soup is anything but, with a zestiness to make a Sicilian proud. What's immediately noticeable is the introduction of tomato into the soup, which makes it almost stewlike when combined with carrots, onions, celery, and a slew of spices. If you're a little under the weather and your sinuses are clogged, they won't be by the time you're done eating some of this tasty twist on the old favorite soup. Chicken is high in zinc, which plays a vital role in memory formation.

2 tablespoons extra-virgin olive oil

1 yellow onion, finely chopped

1 carrot, peeled and cut into $1/2$-inch dice

2 stalks celery, chopped

1 large red potato, peeled and cut into $1/2$-inch dice

Sea salt

3 cloves garlic, chopped

$1/2$ teaspoon fennel seeds

$1/2$ teaspoon dried oregano

$1/2$ teaspoon dried thyme

$1/8$ teaspoon red pepper flakes

1 ($14^1/2$-ounce) can diced tomatoes

6 cups Old-Fashioned Chicken Stock (page 46) or store-bought organic stock

2 cups thinly sliced cooked organic chicken

Freshly squeezed lemon juice

2 tablespoons chopped fresh basil

2 tablespoons chopped parsley

Heat the olive oil in a soup pot over medium-high heat. Add the onion, carrot, celery, potato, and $1/4$ teaspoon of salt and sauté until the vegetables begin to soften, 3 to 5 minutes. Stir in the garlic, fennel, oregano, thyme, and red pepper flakes and cook 1 minute. Stir in the tomatoes with their juice and deglaze the pan. Add the stock and bring to a boil. Decrease the heat to low, cover, and simmer for 15 minutes.

Add the chicken and $1/4$ teaspoon of salt to the soup, stirring to combine. Simmer uncovered for 5 minutes. Remove from the heat and stir in $1/2$ teaspoon of lemon juice and the basil and parsley. Taste; you may want to add another squeeze of lemon juice or pinch of salt. Ladle the soup into bowls and serve immediately.

COOK'S NOTE: Use store-bought roasted chicken or leftover chicken, or you can quickly roast some chicken parts while you're making the rest of the soup. Season one bone-in breast and one bone-in thigh with sea salt, freshly ground black pepper, $1/4$ teaspoon fennel seeds, and a pinch of red pepper flakes. Set the chicken on some sprigs of fresh thyme and bake at 400°F for 25 to 30 minutes. Remove from the oven, allow the chicken to cool, and then cut into bite-size pieces and add to the soup.

PER SERVING: Calories: 221; Total Fat: 10 g (2 g saturated, 6 g mono-unsaturated); Carbohydrates: 15.5 g; Protein: 16 g; Fiber: 3 g; Sodium: 267 mg

STORAGE: Store in an airtight container in the refrigerator for up to 5 days or in the freezer for up to 2 months.

Provençal Seafood Stew

MAKES 4 SERVINGS · PREP TIME: 10 minutes · COOK TIME: 30 minutes

All hail the hearty halibut! That's the song you'll be singing after you try out this stew. Many people avoid halibut because they don't think of it as a tasty fish, but all it needs is the right accompaniments. That's exactly what it gets in this savory French stew, which is rich in aromatics including fennel, leek, and thyme. People equate French food with overly rich Parisian fare, but dishes from the Provence region are much closer to their Mediterranean (that is, healthier) kin. Topping the stew with Parsley Pistou (page 175) got me a sitting ovation from the assembled crew (hey, they would have stood, but they already had their napkins spread over their laps). In the restaurant world, we would call this stew a "well-appointed dish." In my house, we just call it "wow!"

Heat the olive oil in a 4- to 5-quart pot over medium-high heat. Add the leek, shallot, fennel, carrot, and 1/4 teaspoon of salt and sauté until the vegetables begin to soften, 3 to 5 minutes. Stir in the garlic, thyme, and fennel seed. Add the wine and cook for 1 minute. Stir in the tomatoes with their juice and deglaze the pan. Add the broth and bring to a boil. Decrease the heat to low, cover, and simmer for 15 minutes.

Gently stir in the fish and shrimp and simmer until the seafood is tender and cooked through (it should be just opaque), about 4 minutes.

Add the lemon zest, black pepper, and parsley. Taste; you may want to add a pinch or two of sea salt. To serve, ladle the soup into bowls, garnish each with a spoonful of parsley pistou, and serve immediately.

COOK'S NOTE: The pistou takes this soup to the next level; however, if you don't have time to make it, here's a shortcut: garnish with 1/4 cup of chopped parsley, 1 teaspoon of lemon zest, and a spritz of lemon juice.

PER SERVING: Calories: 305; Total Fat: 5.5 g (1 g saturated, 2.5 g monounsaturated); Carbohydrates: 20 g; Protein: 39 g; Fiber: 4 g; Sodium: 715 mg

STORAGE: STORAGE: Store in an airtight container in the refrigerator for up to 3 days.

2 teaspoons extra-virgin olive oil

1 large leek, diced small

1 shallot, diced small

1 fennel bulb, diced small

1 carrot, peeled and diced small

Sea salt

2 cloves garlic, minced

2 teaspoons fresh thyme, or 1/4 teaspoon dried

1/2 teaspoon fennel seed

1/4 cup dry white wine

1 (14 1/2-ounce) can diced tomatoes

3 cups Classic Magic Mineral Broth (page 44) or Old-Fashioned Chicken Stock (page 46), or store-bought organic stock

1 pound halibut fillet, cut into 1 1/2-inch pieces

1 pound large shrimp, peeled and deveined

1/2 teaspoon lemon zest

1/8 teaspoon cracked black pepper

1 tablespoon chopped parsley

Parsley Pistou (page 175), for garnish

Robust Chicken Soup

MAKES 6 SERVINGS • PREP TIME: 20 minutes • COOK TIME: 25 minutes

I'm not sure what I should call this dish. It's more than a soup, but not quite a stew. Maybe it's a stoup (you're laughing now, but just wait till "stoup" makes its way into the Oxford English Dictionary—take that, mochaccino). Well, no matter what you call it, I think you'll find yourself singing its praises often, as this is really a hearty, yummy recipe. This is an instance where putting everything into a simmering broth rather than onto a plate lets some culinary alchemy take place. The result is a feast for the mouth and a source of soothing warmth for the body. This is one of my favorite soups to make when I have leftover chicken in the fridge.

2 cups cooked cannellini beans, or 1 (15-ounce) can, rinsed

Freshly squeezed lemon juice

Sea salt

2 tablespoons extra-virgin olive oil

1 yellow onion, finely diced

2 fennel bulbs, finely diced

2 large carrots, peeled and finely diced

4 stalks celery, finely chopped

2 cloves garlic, minced

$3/4$ teaspoon chopped fresh sage, or $1/4$ teaspoon dried

1 tablespoon fresh thyme leaves, or $1/4$ teaspoon dried

6 cups Old-Fashioned Chicken Stock (page 46) or Classic Magic Mineral Broth (page 44), or store-bought organic stock

2 cups sliced cooked organic chicken

1 teaspoon lemon zest

2 cups arugula leaves

2 tablespoons finely chopped parsley

2 tablespoons finely chopped basil

In a bowl, stir together the beans with a spritz of lemon juice and a pinch of salt. Set aside. Heat the olive oil in a soup pot over medium heat, then add the onion, fennel, carrots, celery, and $1/4$ teaspoon of salt, and sauté until golden, about 15 minutes. Stir in the garlic, sage, and thyme and cook for another minute. Pour in $1/2$ cup of the stock to deglaze the pot, stirring to loosen any bits stuck to the pot, and cook until the liquid is reduced by half. Add the remaining $5^1/2$ cups of stock, the beans, and the chicken, bring to a boil over medium heat, then lower the heat and simmer until the vegetables are tender and the beans and chicken are heated through, about 8 minutes. Stir in the zest, 1 tablespoon of lemon juice, arugula, parsley, basil, and another $1/4$ teaspoon of salt, and serve right away.

VARIATION: Spinach or kale cut into bite-size pieces can be substituted for the arugula.

PER SERVING: Calories: 296; Total Fat: 11 g (2 g saturated, 6 g mono-unsaturated); Carbohydrates: 29 g; Protein: 21 g; Fiber: 9 g; Sodium: 362 mg

STORAGE: Store in an airtight container in the refrigerator for up to 5 days or in the freezer for up to 2 months.

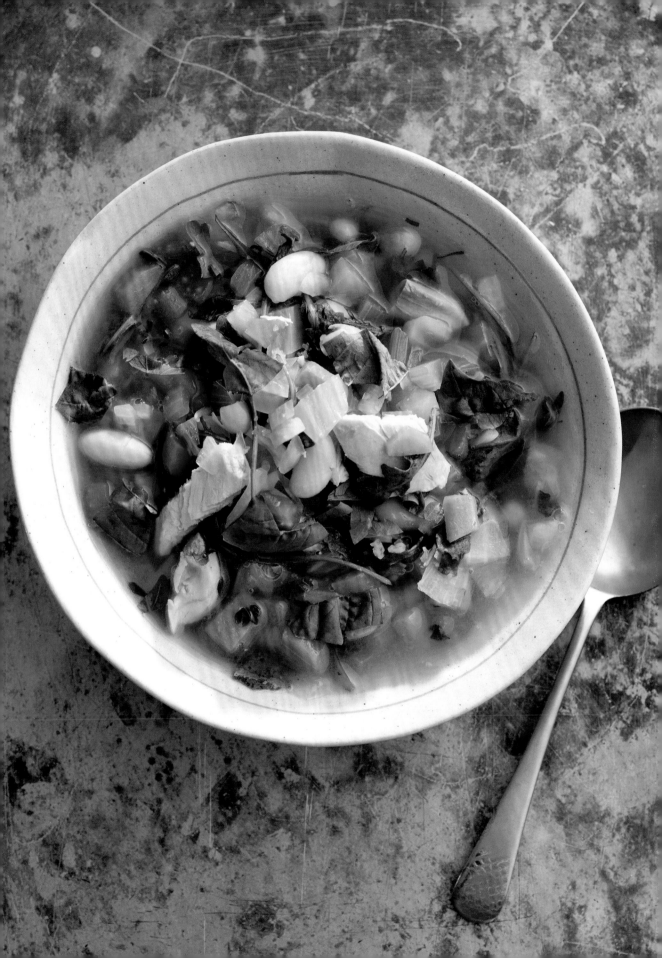

High-Flying Turkey Black Bean Chili

MAKES 6 SERVINGS • PREP TIME: 20 minutes • COOK TIME: 35 minutes

I'll admit it; I'm a bit obsessive when it comes to chili. Most people have one chili powder blend in their pantry. I have four, all of which I buy online at wholespice.com: Chili Powder Dark; ancho chili powder; Chili California Powder; and Chili New Mexico Powder. You get the idea. But my recipe tester Catherine was having none of it when I suggested this recipe include all four of my chili powder blends. "No," she said. "I have one blend, just like any other normal person. Either this is going test well with one blend, or it's not going to fly at all." Fortunately, it achieved the correct flying altitude with just one blend—whichever one you happen to have on hand—but if you want all three (I can't resist), look at the Cook's Note. I love this chili straight up, topped with avocado-cilantro cream, while Catherine likes it best topped with poached eggs. Talk about a protein hit! And for a brain boost, there's nothing like the choline that both black beans and eggs provide.

4 cups cooked black beans, or 2 (15-ounce) cans, rinsed

Freshly squeezed lime juice

Sea salt

3 tablespoons extra-virgin olive oil

1 large yellow onion, chopped

1 large clove garlic, minced

1 jalapeño, deribbed, seeded, and minced

2 teaspoons chili powder

1 teaspoon ancho chile powder

1 teaspoon smoked paprika

1 heaping teaspoon ground cumin

1 teaspoon dried oregano, gently crushed in your hand

1/2 heaping teaspoon ground cinnamon

1 pound ground white or dark turkey meat, or a combination

1 (28-ounce) can crushed tomatoes

In a bowl, combine the drained, rinsed beans with a spritz of lime juice and a pinch of salt; set aside. In a 6-quart pot, heat the olive oil over medium heat. Add the onions and a pinch of salt and sauté for 3 minutes, until the onions are translucent. Add the garlic, jalapeño, chili powder, ancho chile powder, paprika, cumin, oregano, and cinnamon and sauté for another minute. Add the turkey and 1/4 teaspoon of salt, breaking up the meat with a wooden spoon, and brown for about 3 minutes. If the pan is dry or the spices stick, pour in a little juice from the tomatoes to deglaze the pan, stirring with the wooden spoon to loosen any bits stuck to the pan. Add the tomatoes and another pinch of salt, then the peppers and beans and another pinch of salt. Stir to combine. Bring it to a simmer over medium low heat, then cover and simmer for 20 minutes, stirring occasionally.

Remove the cover and simmer for 10 minutes more, stirring occasionally. Stir in the maple syrup. Taste, and add lime juice and salt as needed.

To make the cilantro avocado cream (which is an optional garnish), put the avocado, water, lime juice, cilantro, and salt in a blender and process until very smooth, about 1 minute. Transfer to a small bowl.

Serve the soup in individual bowls garnished with a dollop of the cilantro avocado cream.

COOK'S NOTES: Chili powder is a spice mix made of ground chile peppers (including cayenne), paprika, cumin, garlic, onion, and black pepper. If you use my favorite chili powder blends in this chili, keep the ancho chile powder and, for the 2 teaspoons of chili powder, sub in 2 teaspoons of Chili Dark Powder, 1 teaspoon of Chili New Mexico Powder, and 1 teaspoon of Chili California Powder, all from wholespice.com.

If fresh red bell peppers are not available, jarred roasted red bell peppers will do in a pinch.

If you don't want to haul out your blender or food processor to make the cilantro avocado cream, place all the ingredients in a bowl and mash them together using the back of a fork. It won't be smooth and creamy, but it will still be yummy.

PER SERVING: Calories: 280; Total Fat: 12 g (2 g saturated, 4.25 g mono-unsaturated); Carbohydrates: 29 g; Protein: 20 g; Fiber: 15 g; Sodium: 302 mg

STORAGE: Store in an airtight container in the refrigerator for up to 5 days or in the freezer for up to 2 months.

2 red bell peppers, chopped into bite-size pieces

1 tablespoon Grade B maple syrup

Freshly squeezed lime juice

CILANTRO AVOCADO CREAM (OPTIONAL)

1 avocado, halved and flesh scooped out

2 tablespoons water

3/4 teaspoon freshly squeezed lime juice

2 teaspoons coarsely chopped fresh cilantro

1/4 teaspoon sea salt

Italian Wedding Soup
WITH QUINOA TURKEY MEATBALLS

MAKES 6 SERVINGS · PREP TIME: 15 minutes · COOK TIME: 25 minutes

It's funny how soups get their names. The story I always heard about Italian wedding soup was that it had a lot of pizazz in order to impart some heat to the bride and groom for their impending nookie. It turns out that the Italian got mistranslated: it's not Italian *wedding* soup, but Italian *married* soup. So be it. This version will keep some verve in your swerve. Aromatics set the pace: thyme, oregano, and a wonderful brain-booster, sage, kick up the love. The greens come from shredded cabbage and kale added to the soup and lightly wilted. The soup overall is a magnesium blast, leading us to one Italian word that's never mistranslated: *mangia!*

2 tablespoons extra-virgin olive oil

1 small yellow onion, diced small

Sea salt

3 carrots, peeled and cut into 1/2-inch dice

4 stalks celery, diced

2 cloves garlic, minced

1/2 teaspoon dried thyme

1/2 teaspoon dried oregano

1/2 teaspoon fennel seed

1/4 teaspoon ground sage

8 cups Old-Fashioned Chicken Stock (page 46) or store-bought organic chicken stock

Quinoa Turkey Meatball mixture (page 116)

2 cups finely chopped cabbage

1 cup coarsely chopped, tightly packed dinosaur kale or escarole, or well-chopped curly kale

2 tablespoons coarsely chopped fresh parsley

Heat the olive oil in a soup pot over medium heat. Add the onion and a pinch of salt and sauté until translucent, about 4 minutes. Add the carrots, celery, garlic, thyme, oregano, fennel seed, sage, and 1/4 teaspoon of salt and sauté for about 3 minutes. Add 1/2 cup of the stock to deglaze the pot, stirring to loosen any bits stuck to the pot, and simmer until the liquid is reduced by half. Add the remaining stock, increase the heat to high, and bring to a boil. Decrease the heat to medium-low, cover, and simmer until the vegetables begin to get tender, about 10 minutes.

Use a melon baller or tablespoon to scoop out 24 to 30 balls of the turkey meatball mixture and gently lower them into the broth; make sure they're not too crowded in the pot. Cover and maintain a very gentle simmer so the meatballs don't fall apart as they poach in the soup. After about 4 minutes, add the cabbage and kale. Cook for until the meatballs are cooked all the way through, about another 6 minutes. Stir in the parsley and serve right away.

VARIATION: For a vegetarian dish, substitute 2 cups of cooked cannellini beans for the meatballs. You can use a 15-ounce can of cannellini beans, but be sure to give them the spa treatment: drain, rinse well, and then mix them with a spritz of lemon juice and a pinch of sea salt.

COOK'S NOTE: When you add the meatballs, the temperature of the soup will drop, so you'll need to increase the heat back to a gentle simmer to thoroughly cook the meatballs.

PER SERVING: Calories: 138; Total Fat: 6g (1 g saturated, 4 g monounsaturated); Carbohydrates: 18 g; Protein: 4 g; Fiber: 4 g; Sodium: 153 mg

STORAGE: Store in an airtight container in the refrigerator for up to 5 days or in the freezer for up to 2 months.

Nourishing Beef Bone Broth

MAKES 6 QUARTS • PREP TIME: 25 minutes • COOK TIME: 8 to 16 hours

Beef broth has long been used as a healing tonic, either as the base for soups or as a calming sipping tea. Beef bones are filled with collagen and minerals the body uses to build connective tissues, such as calcium, magnesium, and phosphorus. It also supports healthy digestion, which is important, since what's good for the gut is good for the brain.

Preheat the oven to 425°F.

Place the bones on a baking sheet or roasting pan and roast until the bones are well browned, about 30 minutes.

In a 12-quart or larger stockpot, combine the bones, carrots, onions, celery, garlic, parsley, peppercorns, bay leaves, thyme, and vinegar. Pour in the water, cover, and bring to a boil.

Remove the lid, decrease the heat to low, and skim off the scum that has risen to the top. Simmer gently, uncovered, for 8 to 16 hours.

As the broth simmers, some of the water will evaporate; add more if the vegetables begin to peek out.

Remove and discard the bones, then strain the broth through a large, coarse-mesh sieve. Let cool to room temperature, and then refrigerate overnight. Skim off as much fat as you can from the top of the broth, then portion into airtight containers and refrigerate or freeze.

3 pounds marrow bones from grass-fed organic beef

3 unpeeled carrots, cut into thirds

2 unpeeled yellow onions, cut into chunks

1 bunch celery, including the heart, cut into thirds

5 unpeeled cloves garlic, smashed

1/2 bunch fresh flat-leaf parsley

12 black peppercorns

2 bay leaves

4 sprigs of thyme

1 tablespoon apple cider vinegar

8 quarts cold, filtered water

PER SERVING: Serving Size: 1 cup; Calories: 50; Total Fat: 0 g (0 g saturated, 0 g monounsaturated); Carbohydrates: 11 g; Protein: 1 g; Fiber: 2 g; Sodium: 140 mg

STORAGE: Store in an airtight container in the refrigerator for up to 5 days or in the freezer for up to 4 months.

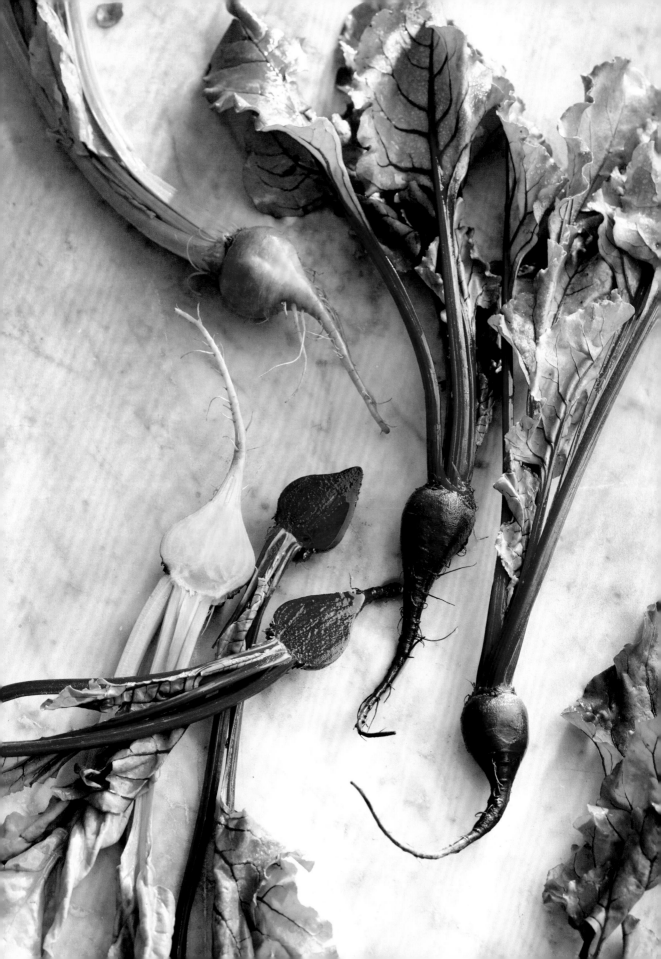

CHAPTER 5

Vegetables

For over a decade, I've been preaching that you need to love your vegetables, not just endure them. Veggies, and the fantastic array of vitamins, minerals, and phytochemicals they contain, are crucial for brain health. For example, cruciferous vegetables (including broccoli, kale, cabbage, and cauliflower) contain B vitamins that are critical for methylation, a process through which our brains repair themselves. Learning to embrace vegetables comes down to flavor and creativity; that's my way of saying that the odds are you grew up on flavorless, drab vegetables that had been boiled within an inch of their lives. But it doesn't have to be that way. In and of themselves, vegetables have wonderful flavor, especially when they're sautéed or roasted, as you'll find in many of the recipes in this chapter.

Many veggies are naturally sweet (like carrots—see Roasted Orange Sesame Carrots on page 93) or savory (see Broccoli with Olives and Lemon Zest on page 90); those that tend to have more of a bite can have their bitterness balanced out by creative pairing with other vegetables (see Kale with Delicata Squash and Hazelnuts, page 84) or fruits (see Orange Salad with Olives and Mint, page 81). Nearly every one of these dishes also has either herbs or spices (or both), as science is showing more and more that these power-packed flavor carriers also carry great brain-boosting properties. Start cooking these recipes and I promise you and your family will never look at veggies the same way again.

Avocado Citrus Salad

MAKES 4 SERVINGS • PREP TIME: 15 Minutes • COOK TIME: 2 to 4 minutes, for variations 15 minutes

There's fat, good fat, and great fat. Avocados fall into the last category—full of brain-boosting vitamin E and a monounsaturated fat that helps lower blood pressure, which can help lower the risk of cognitive impairment. The same fat also serves to signal the gut and brain that satiation is taking place, which keeps us from overeating. In this delicate salad, the avocado acts as a creamy bass note for the tart pop of the grapefruit and the perky citrus-ginger vinaigrette.

1 medium grapefruit or blood orange

Freshly squeezed grapefruit juice

1 teaspoon lemon zest

1 tablespoon freshly squeezed lemon juice

1 tablespoon freshly squeezed lime juice

1 tablespoon honey

1 teaspoon grated ginger

Sea salt

$1/4$ cup extra-virgin olive oil

4 cups loosely packed arugula or mixed greens

$1/2$ cup shaved fennel or celery

$1/4$ cup fresh mint leaves, chopped

1 avocado, sliced

Supreme the grapefruit (see Cook's Note, page 81). When all the segments are out, squeeze the remaining juice into a small bowl and add more grapefruit juice as needed to make 2 tablespoons. Add the zest, lemon juice, lime juice, honey, ginger, and $1/4$ teaspoon of salt and stir to combine. Slowly pour in the olive oil, whisking all the while, and continue whisking until smooth. Transfer to a small container with a fitted lid and shake well.

Mix the arugula, fennel, and mint in a large bowl. Add a tablespoon or two of the dressing and toss. Top with the avocado and grapefruit segments and drizzle with a little more dressing and a light sprinkle of salt.

VARIATIONS: Make this salad heartier by adding grilled shrimp or salmon. Coat 8 ounces of peeled, deveined shrimp or salmon fillet with olive oil and sprinkle with salt. On a grill or in a grill pan, cook over medium high heat until just cooked and opaque, about 2 minutes for shrimp or 3 to 4 minutes for salmon.

COOK'S NOTE: Oranges or tangerines will make a lovely substitution for the grapefruit.

PER SERVING: Calories: 307; Total Fat: 22 g (3 g saturated, 16 g mono-unsaturated); Carbohydrates: 21 g; Protein: 10 g; Fiber: 8 g; Sodium: 345 mg

STORAGE: Store in an airtight container in the refrigerator for up 1 week.

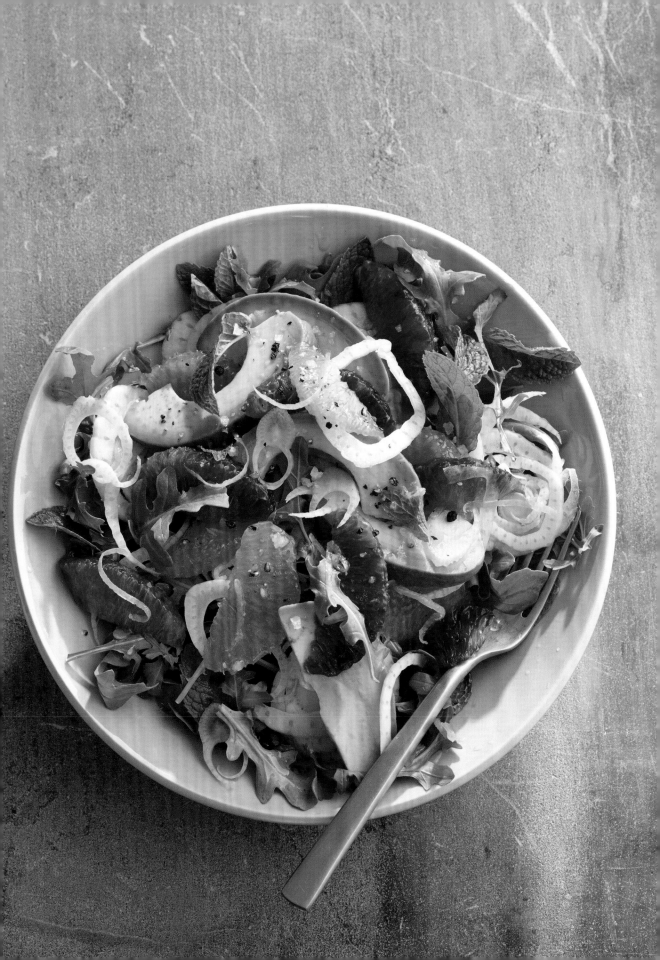

Arugula Salad with Roasted Cherries
AND GOAT CHEESE

MAKES 4 SERVINGS • PREP TIME: 10 minutes • COOK TIME: 5 minutes

Cherries are like Houdini; here one minute, disappeared the next. They have a short summer growing season, no more than two months, so you need to make the most of them when they show their cute, plump selves. Here, I'm playing the sweetness of the cherries off the peppery freshness of arugula, with the bite of goat cheese and balsamic vinegar providing a delightful high note. You don't have to be a Houdini to make these goodies vanish; just bring your appetite.

12 cherries, pitted and halved

1 teaspoon extra-virgin olive oil

Pinch of sea salt

4 cups tightly packed baby arugula

1 cup thinly sliced fennel

2 tablespoons chopped fresh parsley

6 tablespoons Meyer Lemon Balsamic Vinaigrette (page 172)

1/4 cup sliced almonds, toasted

1/4 cup goat cheese (optional)

Preheat the oven to 400°F. Line a baking sheet with parchment paper.

In a bowl, toss the cherries with the olive oil and salt. Place the cherry halves cut side down on the prepared baking sheet and roast for 5 to 6 minutes, until they just begin to soften.

Put the arugula, fennel, warm cherries, and parsley in a large bowl and toss gently to combine. Drizzle the vinaigrette over the top and toss again. Scatter the almonds and goat cheese over, and serve.

VARIATIONS: Substitute toasted walnuts for the almonds.

If cherries are out of season, skip the roasting and use 1 cup of blueberries.

COOK'S NOTE: A mandoline (not to be confused with a mandolin, which is a stringed musical instrument) is a handy kitchen tool that allows you to slice vegetables to a uniform thickness; it's perfect for the fennel in this recipe, which needs to be sliced very thinly. There are many inexpensive models available at kitchen stores and online.

PER SERVING: Calories: 203; Total Fat: 17 g (4 g saturated, 11 g mono-unsaturated); Carbohydrates: 9.5 g; Protein: 5 g; Fiber: 2.5 g; Sodium: 240 mg

STORAGE: Store in an airtight container in the refrigerator for up to 2 days.

Technicolor Slaw

MAKES 4 SERVINGS · PREP TIME: 10 minutes · COOK TIME: Not applicable

I know quite a few cooks (including myself) who like to paint, and when you think about it, that makes sense. We enjoy creating dishes in part because of the ways colors combine to enhance enjoyment of a meal—and, I would argue, also engage the sense of taste. And so it goes here, where the full color palette of food is on display: orange, purple, greens, yellows—it's like Pixar on the plate. Beets are the power player here; they contain natural nitrates, which the body turns into nitric oxide, which in turn expands the walls of blood vessels and increases blood and oxygen flow to benefit the brain and other parts of the body. (The Romans used beets as an aphrodisiac. Enough said.)

Combine the carrots, beet, and raisins in a shallow serving bowl and toss with a pinch of salt. Drizzle in the dressing and toss until evenly coated. Top with the pistachios and mint before serving.

PER SERVING: Calories: 136; Total Fat: 9 g (1 g saturated, 1g monounsaturated); Carbohydrates: 13 g; Protein: 5 g; Fiber: 3 g; Sodium: 226 mg

STORAGE: Store in an airtight container in the refrigerator for up to 2 days.

1 carrots, peeled and shredded

1 red beet, peeled and shredded

2 tablespoons raisins

Generous pinch of sea salt

3 tablespoons Lemon Tahini Dressing (page 181)

2 tablespoons pistachios, toasted

2 tablespoons chopped mint

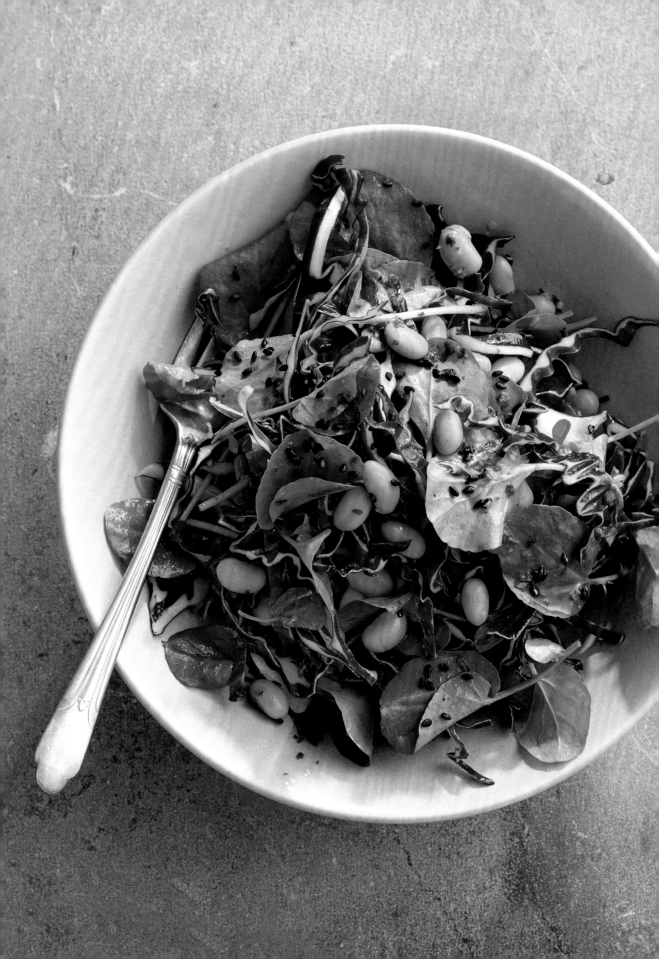

Watercress, Purple Cabbage, and Edamame Salad
WITH TOASTED SESAME SEEDS

MAKES 4 SERVINGS • PREP TIME: 10 minutes • COOK TIME: Not applicable

Cooking sometimes defies math—or, as we're fond of saying around my house, the whole of a dish is often greater than the sum of the parts. Edamame, watercress, cabbage: in themselves, they're a tad less than exciting. Yet when you combine them and add zinc-filled sesame seeds and a cilantro-lime vinaigrette, suddenly you have a salad that's clean, green, and lean. I love it with fish (especially salmon), but it also works well on its own, notably on those days when your body and mind are yearning for culinary refreshment. This would be a great accompaniment to Wild Salmon Kebabs with Asian Pesto (page 112).

Rinse the edamame well and mix with a spritz of lemon juice and a pinch of sea salt. Combine with watercress and cabbage. Dress with the vinaigrette just before serving. Top with sesame seeds and serve immediately.

COOK'S NOTE: To shred cabbage without resorting to a food processor, put the cabbage on a cutting board with the stem side down. Using a sharp chef's knife, cut it in half from top to bottom, then use the tip of the knife to remove the core. Put the halves on the cutting board flat side down and cut in half again. Now you have manageable pieces that you can cut into very thin slices.

PER SERVING: Calories: 163; Total Fat: 14.25 g (1.5 g saturated, 9.7 g monounsaturated); Carbohydrates: 8 g; Protein: 3.75 g; Fiber: 2.25 g; Sodium: 85 mg

STORAGE: This salad does not store well when dressed, but you can refrigerate undressed portions up to 3 days.

1 cup frozen shelled edamame, thawed

Freshly squeezed lemon juice

Sea salt

2 cups tightly packed watercress

2 cups shredded purple cabbage

1/3 cup Cilantro Lime Vinaigrette (page 166)

2 teaspoons sesame seeds, toasted

End of Summer Salad

WITH WATERMELON AND CHERRY TOMATOES

MAKES 4 SERVINGS • PREP TIME: 10 minutes • COOK TIME: 1 MINUTE

Languid days, firefly twilights: this salad just yearns to be made when the calendar hits July and refreshment needs to be close at hand. This quenching dish is an homage to the fruits of summer (and the herbs as well), with watermelon and tomatoes combining with mint to form its heart. Both watermelon and tomatoes are loaded with lycopene, a top-notch antioxidant that protects the brain's high fat content. Lycopene may also play a role in the growth of the brain. A little lime juice and cilantro provide a nice high note for this salad, playing well off the slightly briny creaminess of the feta cheese. All you need is a deck and a hammock and you'll be good to go.

3 cups watermelon, cut into 1-inch pieces

1 cup halved cherry tomatoes

2 tablespoons coarsely chopped mint

2 tablespoons coarsely chopped cilantro

2 tablespoons lime juice

1 teaspoon lime zest

1 tablespoon extra-virgin olive oil

$1/8$ teaspoon freshly ground black pepper

$1/4$ teaspoon sea salt or fleur de sel

$1/4$ cup crumbled feta cheese (optional)

1 tablespoon pumpkin seeds, toasted

Combine the watermelon, tomatoes, mint, cilantro, lime juice and zest, olive oil, and black pepper in a bowl and toss lightly with a fork. Stir in the salt just before serving. Top with the feta and pumpkin seeds and serve.

PER SERVING: Calories: 103; Total Fat: 7 g (2 g saturated, 3 g mono-unsaturated); Carbohydrates: 9 g; Protein: 3 g; Fiber: 1 g; Sodium: 208 mg

STORAGE: This is best eaten the same day it's made. Store in an airtight container in the refrigerator up to 1 day.

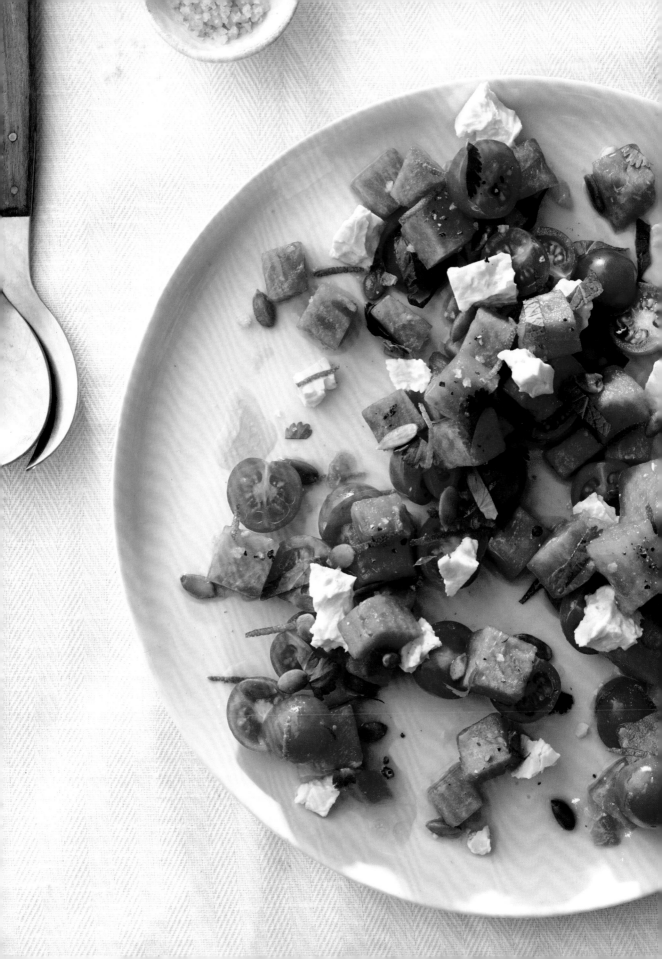

Lentil Salad with Roasted Beets
AND TOASTED CUMIN CITRUS VINAIGRETTE

MAKES 4 SERVINGS • PREP TIME: 20 minutes • COOK TIME: 1 hour

Back in the days when I was a kitchen serf, I received a great piece of culinary advice from a cook. She said to take a food you wanted to work with and imagine preparing it thirty different ways. That's a mental exercise that has served me well over the years, because certain foods are so valuable from a health perspective that they need to show up time and again in new and interesting forms. So it is with lentils. They're so versatile, and they act as a great backdrop for salads and side dishes. In this recipe, they're the foundation for a wonderful blend of citrus and crunch, with fennel, sweet roasted beets, and walnuts all gleefully playing together in the sandbox. Now I just have to come up with twenty-nine more lentil combinations to satisfy that cook.

2 beets

1 cup dried lentils, preferably Le Puy green lentils, rinsed well

1 clove garlic, peeled and smashed

1 bay leaf

1 cinnamon stick, or $1/4$ teaspoon ground cinnamon

$1/2$ cup Toasted Cumin Citrus Vinaigrette (page 170)

Sea salt

1 cup diced fennel

3 tablespoons chopped fresh mint

3 tablespoons chopped flat-leaf parsley

$1/4$ cup walnuts, toasted and coarsely chopped

Freshly squeezed lemon juice

Freshly ground black pepper

Preheat the oven to 425°F. Wrap the beets in parchment paper, then in foil, and roast for 30 minutes to 1 hour (depending on their size), until tender and fragrant. Remove from the oven and, when they are cool enough, peel and cut into small cubes.

Combine the lentils, garlic, bay leaf, and cinnamon in a saucepan and cover with water by 2 inches. Bring to a boil, then cover, lower the heat, and simmer until the lentils are tender, 20 to 25 minutes. Drain the lentils thoroughly and discard the garlic clove, bay leaf, and cinnamon stick.

Toss the lentils with half the vinaigrette and $1/4$ teaspoon of salt and let it rest a few minutes. Then add the fennel, beets, and remaining dressing. Stir in the mint and parsley, walnuts, and a teaspoon of lemon juice. Taste; you may want to add another pinch of salt, a few grinds of black pepper, or a bit more lemon juice. Serve.

VARIATION: This salad can also be heated and served over arugula or spinach. The heat will gently wilt the greens.

COOK'S NOTE: You don't have to presoak lentils, but rinse them well in a bowl of cold water, using your hands to swish them around. Drain and repeat until the water is clear. Don't boil lentils, which makes them mushy and causes them to fall apart. Let them simmer for a nice, tender texture.

PER SERVING: Calories: 268; Total Fat: 15 g (1.8 g saturated, 9 g mono-unsaturated); Carbohydrates: 27 g; Protein: 9.5 g; Fiber: 8.5 g; Sodium: 77.5 mg

STORAGE: Store in an airtight container in the refrigerator for up to 4 days.

Italian White Bean Salad

MAKES 4 SERVINGS · PREP TIME: 10 minutes · COOK TIME: Not applicable

Often when I'm developing a recipe, I think about texture as much as taste. That is the case here, where there's a creamy/crunchy thing going between the white beans and the radishes. This is the kind of light fare Italians are known for and that I commonly found served up as antipasti as I traveled across that country. Olives, scallions, mint, and parsley round out the salad, which is tossed in a traditional Italian salsa verde. Radishes, which create a great mouthfeel, are a brassica, which means they have lots of brain-boosting properties including regulating blood sugar.

In a large bowl, stir together the cannellini beans, a spritz of lemon, and a pinch of salt. Add the salsa verde and stir to coat the beans. Add the radishes, olives, parsley, scallions, and mint and toss. Taste; you may want to give it a squeeze of lemon or another pinch or two of salt. Serve.

COOK'S NOTE: Cannellini beans will soak up the salsa verde, so if you want to store this salad in the refrigerator, perk it up with another teaspoon of dressing or a spritz of lemon.

PER SERVING: Calories: 264; Total Fat: 17 g (2.5 g saturated, 13.5g monounsaturated); Carbohydrates: 21.5 g; Protein: 8.5 g; Fiber: 7 g; Sodium: 653 mg

STORAGE: Store in an airtight container in the refrigerator for up to 3 days.

2 cups cooked cannellini beans, or 1 (15-ounce) can, rinsed

Freshly squeezed lemon juice

Sea salt

$^1/_2$ cup Signora Francini's Salsa Verde (page 174)

6 radishes, quartered and cut into $^1/_4$ inch pieces

12 kalamata olives, pitted and sliced

$^1/_2$ cup coarsely chopped fresh parsley

2 scallions, sliced

2 tablespoons chopped fresh mint

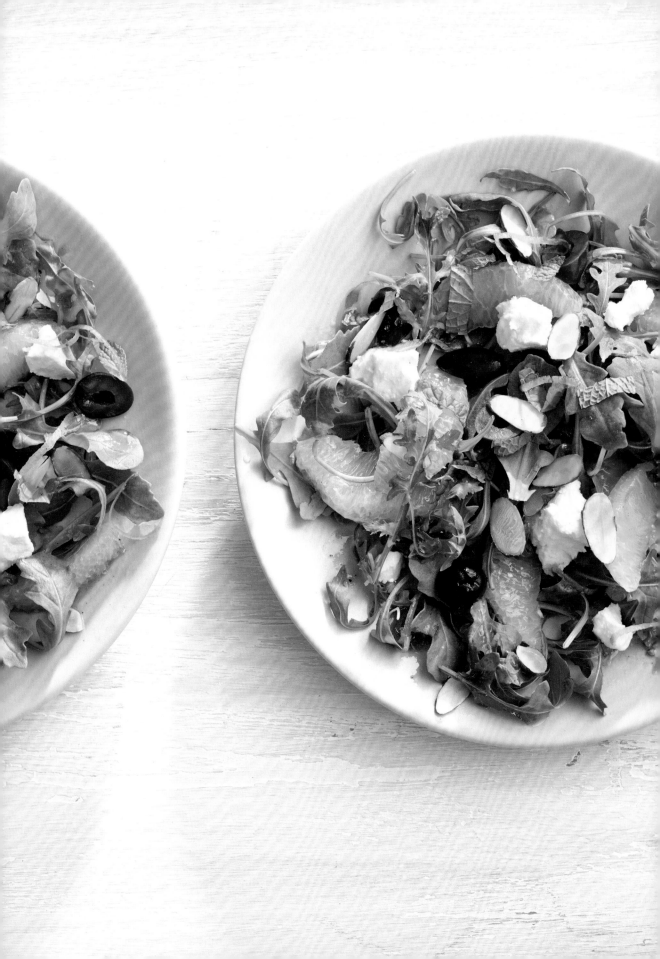

Orange Salad with Olives and Mint

MAKES 4 SERVINGS · PREP TIME: 20 minutes · COOK TIME: Not applicable

One of the great things about traveling is that it gets you out of food ruts. When you're in a different part of the country, or of the world, it's hard to ignore local fare. When an eighty-year-old *nonna* puts a strange salad in front of you, what are you going to say—"No?" I remember the first time I saw this salad in Italy. My initial reaction was, "Oranges with cracked pepper? Really?!" And yet this combination, and another one I saw with oranges and olives, really kicked up an incredible sweet-salty mouth pop that was impossible to ignore. Clearly the combo left an impression, because I've reprised it here with my own touch, adding almonds and mint. Maybe it was more than an impression; let's call it inspiration—just the type of culinary experience that primes the pump of creativity.

Put the arugula, oranges, olives, and mint in a large bowl and toss gently to combine. Drizzle the vinaigrette over the top and toss again. Scatter the almonds, a few generous grinds of black pepper, and the goat cheese over the top.

VARIATIONS: Substitute toasted walnuts for the almonds.

Use a variety of oranges, such as Valencias, blood oranges, or tangerines.

COOK'S NOTE: "Supreme" is such a cheffy term. It means cutting the skin and the membrane away from the segments of a citrus fruit. Using a sharp paring knife, trim the bottom of the orange to create a flat surface. Place the orange with the flat surface on your cutting board and trim off the remainder of the skin and white pith, by curving your knife downward in the shape of the fruit's natural shape. Then, segment by segment, slice to the left and right of each membrane, freeing the flesh of each segment from the membrane. Another option is to pare away the skin and white pith, and slice the oranges in circles.

PER SERVING: Calories: 274; Total Fat: 21 g (4.5 g saturated, 16.5 g monounsaturated); Carbohydrates: 14 g; Protein: 4.5 g; Fiber: 3 g; Sodium: 422 mg

STORAGE: Not applicable

4 cups tightly packed baby arugula or mixed greens

2 oranges, supremed (see Cook's Note)

12 pitted kalamata olives, rinsed and sliced

3 tablespoons chopped fresh mint

4 tablespoons Orange Pomegranate Vinaigrette (page 171)

2 tablespoons sliced almonds, toasted

Freshly ground black pepper

2 ounces goat cheese, crumbled (optional)

Kale with Dates
AND CARAMELIZED ONIONS

MAKES 6 SERVINGS · PREP TIME: 10 minutes · COOK TIME: 15 minutes

I never thought I'd see the day, but kale has become the "in" vegetable—at least here on the West Coast. It's a far cry from the days when people would look at a bundle of kale like it was a shrub, and make whining noises at the thought of turning it into a meal. So what's changed? Two things. First, it's hard to look at kale's incredible nutritional profile and *not* want to get it into your diet. Just a cup of kale contains 90 percent of all the vitamin C you need in a day; one study showed loading up on these kinds of antioxidants reduced cognitive impairment in an elderly population. Second, people got exposed to enough creative and delicious kale dishes to want to tackle it themselves. With a little creativity, kale can be a centerpiece for a fine salad, as this recipe shows. This dish is a festival on the plate, with eye-popping colors coming from the ruby pomegranate seeds playing against the greens of the kale and mint.

2 tablespoons extra-virgin olive oil

1 red onion, cut into quarter moons

Sea salt

1 clove garlic, minced

Pinch of red pepper flakes

2 tablespoons chopped dates

2 dinosaur kale, stemmed and chopped into bite-size pieces (see Cook's Note)

Freshly squeezed lemon juice

1 tablespoon pomegranate seeds

In a large, deep sauté pan, heat the olive oil over medium-high heat. Add the onion and a pinch of salt. Sauté for 3 to 5 minutes. Decrease the heat to low and cook slowly until the onions are just caramelized, about 5 minutes more.

Add the garlic and stir for about 30 seconds, just until aromatic. Add the red pepper flakes and dates, and stir for about 30 seconds. Add 2 tablespoons of water to the pan to deglaze it, scraping with a spoon to loosen all the flavorful bits from the bottom of the pan. Add as many greens as will fit to the pan, along with a pinch of salt. The water that adheres to the greens will be enough liquid to wilt them; when they've wilted down enough, add the rest of the greens, if any haven't made it into the pan yet. Taste the greens, add an additional tablespoon of water if needed, cover the pan, and cook until the greens are tender, 2 to 3 minutes. Add 2 teaspoons of lemon juice and taste again, adding of pinch of salt or another spritz of lemon juice, if necessary.

Arrange the greens on plates and sprinkle the pomegranate seeds on top. Serve hot.

COOK'S NOTES: One trick to preparing hearty greens like kale or chard is to rip them off their tough spines. This makes them easier to eat and digest. Once you've stemmed your greens (a great job for the little ones), chop them (the greens, not the kids) into bite-size pieces with your sharp chef's knife. When you add your greens to the pan they will resemble Mount Vesuvius, but you'll be surprised how quickly that volcano of greens shrinks into a small mound.

Another trick for preparing greens is to put them in a bowl of cold water for a bath; this allows dirt and sand to fall to the bottom. Remove the greens from the water, stack the leaves and roll them up, then cut the rolls into thin ribbons, and then lengthwise into small bite-size pieces.

PER SERVING: Calories: 133; Total Fat: 8 g (1 g saturated, 5.5 g mono-unsaturated); Carbohydrates: 16 g; Protein: 4 g; Fiber: 3 g; Sodium: 144 mg

STORAGE: Store in an airtight container in the refrigerator for up to 3 days.

Kale with Delicata Squash
AND HAZELNUTS

MAKES 6 SERVINGS · PREP TIME: 10 minutes · COOK TIME: 20 minutes

Getting in the swing of eating veggies is like igniting a pilot light on a stove: it may take several tries, but once it's lit, the flame burns steadily. My challenge is to present important vegetables—and, none is more vital for brain health than kale—in ways that will kick-start your taste for this superfood. Here, I've paired kale with an autumn favorite, delicata squash, along with garlic, red pepper flakes, and freshly squeezed lemon juice to create a dish that's both a delight to the eyes and the taste buds. The chopped roasted hazelnuts take the entire concoction completely over the top. It's ablaze with flavor and should leave you burning for more.

2 bunches dinosaur kale, stemmed and cut in bite-size pieces (see Cook's Note, page 83)

2 tablespoons extra-virgin olive oil

2 cloves garlic, minced

1/8 teaspoon red pepper flakes

1 medium delicata squash, seeded and flesh cut into bite-size pieces

Sea salt

Freshly squeezed lemon juice

1/4 teaspoon Grade B maple syrup

1/4 cup hazelnuts, toasted and chopped

Cover the kale with cold water and set aside. Heat the olive oil in a large, deep sauté pan over medium heat, then stir in the garlic and red pepper flakes and sauté for about 15 seconds, then immediately add the squash and a pinch of salt. Stir to combine. Let cook until the squash is caramelized and just tender, about 10 minutes.

Drain the kale and add it to the pan in batches along with 1/4 teaspoon salt. Sauté until the greens turn bright green and wilt, about 5 minutes. Test the greens for tenderness; you may need to add 1 tablespoon of water and continue cooking, covered for another 2 to 3 minutes. Drizzle on 1 tablespoon of lemon juice and the maple syrup and stir gently. Taste; you may want to add a pinch or two of salt and another squeeze of lemon. Garnish with the hazelnuts and serve immediately.

PER SERVING: Calories: 134; Total Fat: 8 g (1 g saturated, 6 g monounsaturated); Carbohydrates: 13.5 g; Protein: 4 g; Fiber: 3 g; Sodium: 105 mg

STORAGE: Store in an airtight container in the refrigerator for up to 3 days.

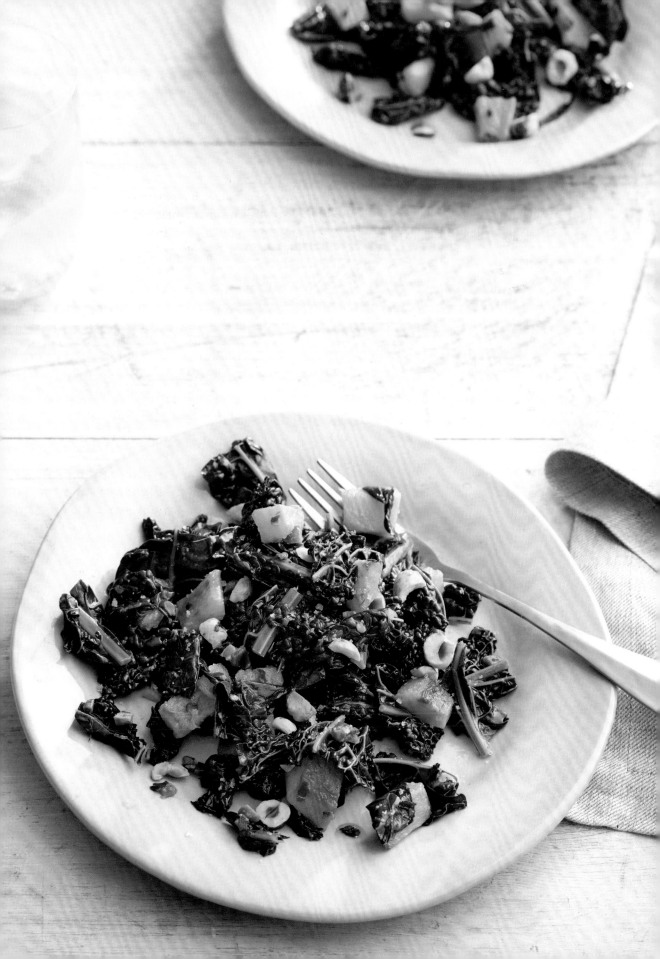

Coconut Ginger Lime Kale

MAKES 4 SERVINGS · PREP TIME: 5 minutes · COOK TIME: 10 minutes

I like to make kale a world traveler; in other books I've managed to stamp its passport with Asian, Latin American, and Mediterranean flavorprints. This time I've booked kale's passage to Thailand, in whose cuisine coconut, ginger, and lime can often be found.

Coconut milk helps increase the bioavailability of kale's fat-soluble vitamins, while coconut's sweetness and the brightness of the lime help eliminate kale's natural bitterness. I've taken kale so many places I'm amazed I don't have Customs showing up at my front door. But if they do, I'll just make them this dish and they'll go away satisfied.

2 tablespoons extra-virgin olive oil or coconut oil

2 cloves garlic, minced

1 tablespoon minced fresh ginger

1 bunch kale, stemmed and cut into bite-size pieces (see page 83)

1/4 teaspoon sea salt

1/2 cup coconut milk

1 1/2 teaspoons freshly squeezed lime juice

Heat the oil in a large pan over medium-high heat. Add the garlic and ginger, stir, and cook about a minute. Add the kale and salt, and sauté for 3 minute or just until it turns an emerald green. Add the coconut milk and sauté continuously until the kale is tender, about 5 minutes. Stir in the lime juice and serve immediately.

VARIATIONS: For some color, add 1/2 cup of finely diced red or yellow bell pepper along with the kale.

If you have Thai basil, garnish with 1 tablespoon, chopped, for a real Asian flare.

PER SERVING: Calories: 142 Total Fat: 11 g (4 g saturated, 6 g mono-unsaturated); Carbohydrates: 11 g; Protein: 4 g; Fiber: 2 g; Sodium: 145 mg

STORAGE: Store in an airtight container in the refrigerator for up to 4 days.

Brandon's Roasted Broccoli

MAKES 4 SERVINGS · PREP TIME: 10 minutes · COOK TIME: 15 minutes

They say kids don't like vegetables, but my grandson Brandon evidently didn't get that memo. He's eaten and loved veggies since the age of two (he's seven now), with broccoli being his favorite. He's not shy about it, either. Last time he was over I asked him how he wanted his broccoli. He said, "Roasted . . . where you lay them out on a cookie sheet." Want a scene that'll melt your heart? That's watching Brandon down on all fours, peering through the glass into the oven at his broccoli baking. When they come out, I put a little Parmesan cheese on top, and Brandon's picking them off the roasting pan.

Position a rack in the middle of the oven and preheat the oven to 400°F. Line a rimmed baking sheet with parchment paper.

Put the broccoli, olive oil, garlic, salt, pepper, and lemon zest in a large bowl and toss until the broccoli is evenly coated. Transfer to the lined baking sheet and spread it in an even layer. Bake for 15 to 20 minutes, until the broccoli begins to brown and is tender.

Transfer to a bowl, add the Parmesan, and basil, and toss to combine. Add the lemon zest and a spritz of lemon juice and serve immediately.

VARIATION: Swap the Parmesan cheese and basil with toasted sesame seeds, and toss with Lemon Tahini Dressing (page 181).

COOK'S NOTE: Be sure to add the lemon juice and zest just before serving, as the lemon will dull the color of the broccoli if it sits for more than a few minutes.

PER SERVING: Calories: 165; Total Fat: 9.5 g (2 g saturated, 6 g mono-unsaturated); Carbohydrates: 16 g; Protein: 10.5 g; Fiber: 9 g; Sodium: 353 mg

STORAGE: Store in an airtight container in the refrigerator for up to 2 days.

2$\frac{1}{2}$ pounds broccoli, cut into florets with 2 inches of trimmed stem

2 tablespoons extra-virgin olive oil

1 tablespoon minced garlic

$\frac{1}{2}$ teaspoon sea salt

$\frac{1}{4}$ teaspoon freshly ground black pepper

$\frac{1}{4}$ cup Parmesan cheese (optional)

1 tablespoon chopped fresh basil (optional)

1 teaspoon lemon zest

Freshly squeezed lemon juice

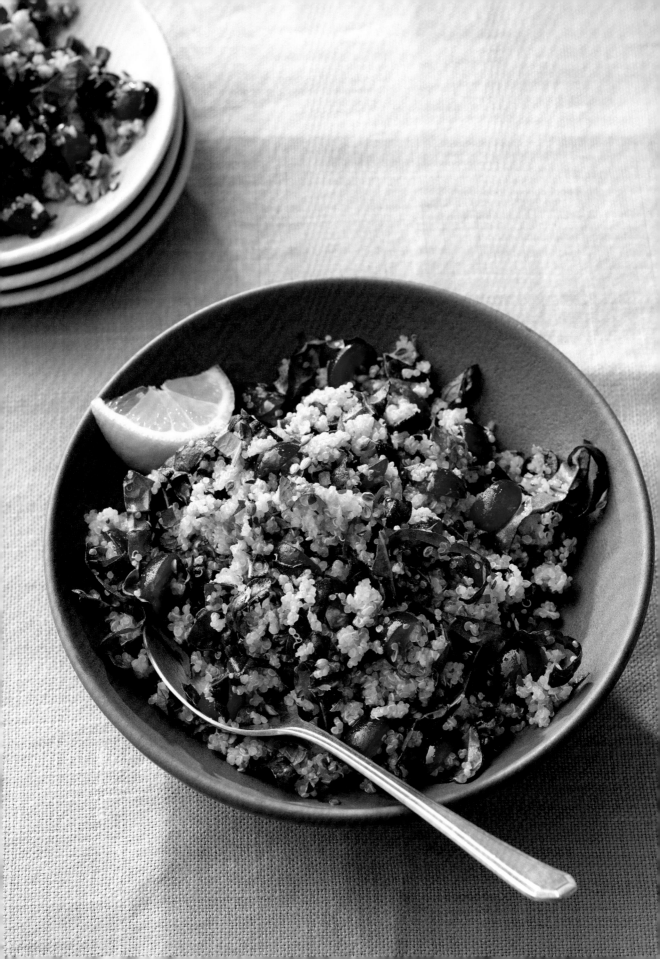

Kale Quinoa Salad
WITH RED GRAPES

MAKES 4 SERVINGS · PREP TIME: 10 minutes · COOK TIME: 20 minutes

Kale is quirky; with the right touch it shines like an emerald and tastes delish, but if you ignore a few key steps it can resemble Astroturf. Fortunately, it doesn't take much to get on kale's good side. Once it's ripped and stripped it loves a bath in olive oil, lemon juice, and salt. This spa treatment break down the kale's fibers, making it easier to digest (the olive oil's fat also increases the bioavailability of kale's fat-soluble nutrients). I've included mint, parsley, quinoa, cumin, and coriander in the dish and added one additional surprise: red grapes. There's something about chomping on a sweet grape that's just joyous, and the anthocyanins that give the grape its deep color are also phenomenal antioxidants, with other studies showing they may also enhance memory.

Place the quinoa in a fine-mesh strainer and rinse well under cold running water.

In a small saucepan, bring 1 1/2 cups of water and 1/2 teaspoon of the salt to a boil over high heat. Add the quinoa and cover. Decrease the heat to low and simmer for 15 to 20 minutes, stirring once halfway through, until the quinoa is just tender. Remove from the heat and allow the quinoa to rest for 10 minutes. Fluff the quinoa with a fork.

While the quinoa is cooking, whisk together the lemon juice, the remaining 1/4 teaspoon of salt, cumin, coriander, red pepper flakes, and olive oil together in a large bowl. Add the kale and give it a quick massage with your hands. Add the quinoa, mint, parsley, lemon zest, and grapes and toss lightly to combine. Serve at room temperature.

COOK'S NOTE: When you make quinoa, rinse it well. Quinoa is naturally coated with a bitter-tasting resin. To get rid of the resin, put the grain in a bowl of cool water, swish it around with your hand, and drain it in a fine-mesh sieve.

PER SERVING: Calories: 281; Total Fat: 16 g (2 g saturated, 11 g mono-unsaturated); Carbohydrates: 32 g; Protein: 6 g; Fiber: 4 g; Sodium: 325 mg

STORAGE: Store in an airtight container in the refrigerator for up to 5 days.

1 cup quinoa

3/4 teaspoon sea salt

1/4 cup freshly squeezed lemon juice

1/2 teaspoon cumin

1/4 teaspoon coriander

Pinch of red pepper flakes

1/2 cup extra-virgin olive oil

2 cups stemmed and finely chopped kale

1/4 cup lightly packed chopped fresh mint,

1/4 cups lightly packed chopped parsley

1 teaspoon lemon zest

1/4 cup halved red seedless grapes, or 3 tablespoons raisins

Broccoli with Olives
AND LEMON ZEST

MAKES 4 SERVINGS · PREP TIME: 10 minutes · COOK TIME: 10 minutes

If kale is now the star of the cruciferous set, I'd still nominate broccoli for a Best Supporting Actor award. Broccoli is so good for the brain—animal studies showed a phytochemical in broccoli, sulforaphane, protected against damage from brain injury—that I consider it a superfood. Broccoli is also loaded with fat-soluble vitamins that benefit from being served with a good fat source, in this case olives. I've long loved olives; in fact, as a kid I used to use my fingers like toothpicks and stick olives on the end of them. Here you don't need fingers, just a sauté pan.

3 tablespoons extra-virgin olive oil

2 cloves garlic, finely chopped

$1/4$ teaspoon dried oregano

$1/8$ teaspoon red pepper flakes

1 bunch of broccoli, cut into florets (about $2^1/2$ cups)

$1/4$ teaspoon sea salt

$1/4$ cup olives, chopped

2 scallions, thinly sliced

2 teaspoons lemon zest

Heat the olive oil in a large sauté pan over medium-high heat. Add the garlic, oregano, and red pepper flakes and sauté just until aromatic, about 30 seconds. Add the broccoli and salt. Sauté until tender and crisp, 7 or 8 minutes. You may need to add 1 to 2 tablespoons of water if the pan gets too dry. The broccoli should still be firm. Stir in the olives, scallions, and lemon zest and serve immediately.

VARIATIONS: Top with chopped toasted almonds or walnuts if you like. Or, for extra brainpower, add two chopped anchovies and 1 teaspoon of rinsed capers just before adding the broccoli.

PER SERVING: Calories: 120; Total Fat: 12 g (2 g saturated, 9 g mono-unsaturated); Carbohydrates: 4 g; Protein: 2 g; Fiber: 2 g; Sodium: 240 mg

STORAGE: Store in an airtight container in the refrigerator for up to 3 days.

Julie's Sweet-and-Sour Cabbage

MAKES 6 SERVINGS · PREP TIME: 15 minutes · COOK TIME: 45 minutes

Making sweet-and-sour anything reminds me of being a kid and sitting on a seesaw with a buddy; if you balance things *just* right, the two of you can both stay in the air indefinitely (and isn't that a cool feeling). But throw off the balance a mere inch, and one of you comes thudding back to earth. So it went the first time I tried making this dish. It's actually my friend Julie's recipe; I sat in her kitchen, furiously scribbling notes as she put this dish together, but somewhere I turned just a touch of ginger into a nuclear blast. Not to fret: names were taken, the usual suspects rounded up, and sanity prevailed. What's left is a sweet-and-sour cabbage that's absolutely addictive.

Shred the cabbage in a food processor or cut the head into quarters and slice it thinly with a knife.

Heat the olive oil in a large sauté pan and sauté the onion and a pinch of salt until translucent, about 6 minutes. Add the cabbage and 1/4 teaspoon of salt and sauté for about 5 minutes.

Add the apple, caraway, 1/2 teaspoon of freshly ground black pepper, and another pinch of salt to the pan and sauté for a minute or two. Pour the red wine into the pan and let it reduce by half. Then add 1/3 cup of water and the vinegar and brown sugar and stir to combine. Reduce the heat to low, cover, and simmer for 30 to 35 minutes, or until tender. Taste; you may want to add a pinch of salt or a few grinds of pepper. Serve.

PER SERVING: Calories: 90; Total Fat: 2.5 g (.5 g saturated, 2 g monounsaturated); Carbohydrates: 15.5 g; Protein: 1 g; Fiber: 2.5 g; Sodium: 85 mg

STORAGE: Store in an airtight container in the refrigerator for up to 1 week.

1 (12-ounce) head red cabbage

1 tablespoon extra-virgin olive oil

1 small yellow onion, finely diced

Sea salt

1 crisp organic apple, finely diced

1 teaspoon caraway seeds

Freshly ground black pepper

1/3 cup full-bodied red wine

3 tablespoons apple cider vinegar

2 tablespoons light brown sugar or coconut palm sugar

My Friend Jo's Special Sauerkraut

MAKES 2 QUART JARS • PREP TIME: 15 minutes • COOK TIME: Up to 10 days

I'll admit it: I'm a ham. Take the last time I demonstrated how to make sauerkraut. The recipe is pretty basic: pulverize some cabbage, pour some salt over it in a crock, cover, and ferment. Not the most exciting of demos—unless you've got a friend, like my friend Jo, with a great sense of humor and knowledge of *moi*. I told her I needed a mallet for the demo; she lent me her mother's mallet. It was about eighty years old and five feet tall, and was so big I had to get on top of a milk crate to wield it. It was chancy—the room was filled with three hundred health care professionals—but we all got a good laugh out of it. Hijinks aside, sauerkraut is easy to make—and it's a great probiotic, leading to a sound gut, which, as scientists are learning, makes for a sound mind.

3 pounds cabbage, shredded

8 ounces carrots, peeled and shredded

3 tablespoons sea salt

1$\frac{1}{2}$ tablespoons coriander seed, gently crushed

In a large bowl, combine the cabbage, carrots, salt, and coriander. Using your hands, crush the mixture together until it starts to release moisture, about 5 minutes. The liquid will begin to pool at the bottom of the bowl. Transfer the cabbage mixture into two new and clean 32-ounce mason jars, packing down the mixture with a spoon or your hand. Pressing it will bring the liquid to the top and release any air bubbles from the bottom. There should be about $\frac{1}{2}$ inch of liquid over the cabbage. Cover with whole cabbage leaves and weigh down the mixture with a clean glass or cup filled with stones or pie weights.

Cover the jar with a linen, cotton, or cheese cloth and secure it with a rubber band. Set the jar in a bowl to catch any liquid that may overflow. Store in a cool, dark place for at least 2 days and up to 7 to 14, depending on the temperature. Taste each day until the tangy flavor is just right, then cover it with a lid and store it in the refrigerator.

COOK'S NOTES: If you use too little salt, the mixture will mold. Too much salt, and it will not ferment. My research shows about 1$\frac{3}{4}$ teaspoons of sea salt per pound of cabbage is a good rule of thumb.

The mixture can ferment on the counter for up to 10 days. A cool room temperature of 64°F is ideal. If it's warmer, check it more often than once a day. You may see bubbles, foam, or white froth on the surface, but these are all signs of normal fermentation. The white froth can be skimmed off as you see it or before refrigerating the sauerkraut.

PER SERVING: Serving Size: $\frac{1}{2}$ cup; Calories: 29; Total Fat: 0 g (0 g saturated, 0 g monounsaturated); Carbohydrates: 6.5 g; Protein: 1 g; Fiber: 3 g; Sodium: 235 mg

STORAGE: Store in an airtight container for up to 2 months.

Roasted Orange Sesame Carrots

MAKES 4 SERVINGS · PREP TIME: 5 minutes · COOK TIME: 40 minutes

One school of thought says that in order to get kids to eat their veggies you have to "hide" them within a meal. Well, I never graduated from that institution. Want a child to love veggies? Serve them these carrots. My cooking buddies and I joke that, though the recipe says "serves 4," it should really say "feeds one," because they're that compelling. This is a great natural sweetness fest, between the carrots, orange, and a drape of organic maple syrup. Hopefully your kids are good at sharing, but don't be surprised if they end up arm wrestling over the last one of these.

Preheat the oven to 400°F. Line two baking sheets with parchment paper.

In a large bowl, whisk together the orange zest and juice, maple syrup, olive oil, and 1/2 teaspoon of salt. Add the carrots and toss to coat. Spread evenly in the two pans, well spaced. Bake for 40 minutes or until tender and caramelized. Sprinkle with sesame seeds and a pinch of salt. Serve immediately.

COOK'S NOTE: If using regular large-size carrots, peel them, quarter them lengthwise, and then cut them in half, as if they were carrot sticks. Make sure the carrots are not crowded together on the pan or they will steam instead of developing that wonderful caramelization that happens to vegetables when they roast.

PER SERVING: Calories: 148; Total Fat: 6 g (1 g saturated, 4 g monounsaturated); Carbohydrates: 23.5 g; Protein: 2 g; Fiber: 7 g; Sodium: 379 mg

STORAGE: Store in an airtight container in the refrigerator for up to 4 days.

1 teaspoon orange zest

3 tablespoons freshly squeezed orange juice

1 tablespoon Grade B maple syrup

1 1/2 tablespoons extra-virgin olive oil

Sea salt

2 pounds small carrots, tops trimmed and cut lengthwise into equal-size pieces

1 teaspoon sesame seeds, toasted

Celery Root Mash-Up

MAKES 4 SERVINGS · PREP TIME: 10 minutes · COOK TIME: 25 minutes

This is a culinary equivalent of the story of the ugly duckling. If you've ever stumbled across a celery root without knowing what it was, your first reaction may have been "get that nasty thing away from me!" It looks like a softball that was played with in the mud for weeks on end. And yet, beneath its exterior, which you can easily hack away, lies the most wonderful, succulent root, which, with just a little work, turns into the most delicious, pearly mash. With a sublime yet gentle taste, celery root makes a fantastic base to blend with other foods, in this case olive oil, capers, and Dijon mustard. Show it the love, and celery root blooms into a beautiful swan right before your eyes. It's also packed with great calming nutrients, including magnesium.

2 pounds celery root, trimmed, peeled, and cut into $1/2$-inch cubes (see Cook's Note)

Sea salt

Classic Magic Mineral Broth (page 44), Old-Fashioned Chicken Stock (page 46), store-bought organic stock, or water

2 tablespoons butter or ghee, or 3 tablespoons extra-virgin olive oil

1 tablespoon capers, rinsed

1 teaspoon Dijon mustard

Freshly squeezed lemon juice

2 tablespoons minced fresh parsley

Put the celery root and a few pinches of salt in a pot and add enough broth or other liquid to cover by 1 inch. Bring to a boil over high heat, then lower the heat to low, cover, and simmer for 20 to 25 minutes, or until the celery root is very tender. Drain in a colander, reserving the cooking water. Transfer the celery root to the bowl of a food processor and add the butter, capers, mustard, $1/4$ teaspoon of salt, and $1/4$ teaspoon of lemon juice. Process until smooth, adding some of the reserved cooking water 1 tablespoon at a time until the desired consistency is achieved. Taste; you may want to add a few pinches of salt and a squeeze of lemon. Add the parsley to the bowl and pulse a few times, until combined. Serve immediately.

VARIATION: For a richer mash, use Almond Milk (page 195) instead of the cooking liquid to thin the mash.

COOK'S NOTE: How do you peel celery root? Place the root on its side. Using a sharp knife, cut off the bottom to create a flat edge. Stand the root upright. Cut the remaining peel off in vertical strips from top to bottom, following the shape of the root until you have removed all of the skin. Rinse the peeled root and cut it into cubes. If you're prepping celery root in advance, place it in a bowl of cold water with a squeeze of lemon to keep it from turning brown.

PER SERVING: Calories: 146; Total Fat: 6 g (4 g saturated, 0.15 g mono-unsaturated); Carbohydrates: 21 g; Protein: 4 g; Fiber: 4 g; Sodium: 426 mg

STORAGE: Store in the refrigerator for up to 2 days.

Rutabaga and Potato Mash-Up

MAKES 6 SERVINGS · PREP TIME: 10 minutes · COOK TIME: 35 minutes

Rutabaga sounds funny unless you're Swedish; it's just their word for turnip. Don't ask me why, but rutabagas were a staple in my house when I was growing up, and I still love them. They've actually changed some over the years; there are now hybrids that cross them with cabbage, creating a slightly sweet flavor. As far as brain boosters go, they're the full package, offering magnesium to reduce stress, manganese for energy, and a load of beta-carotene to lower oxidative damage. For Thanksgiving, my mom would make a version of this flavorful mash, and I'd always walk by, stick my finger in the bowl, and come away with a smile. It only took two generations for this mash to come around on the turntable again, but it's kind of like the Beatles or Elvis: it really never gets old.

Put the rutabaga and $1/4$ teaspoon of salt into a pot and add enough broth or other liquid to cover by 2 inches. Bring to a boil over high heat, then lower the heat to medium-high, cover, and simmer until the rutabagas are tender, 25 to 30 minutes. Add the potatoes to the pot, cover, and let simmer until the potatoes are tender and mashable, about another 10 minutes. Drain in a colander, reserving the cooking water. Transfer the vegetables back to the pot and add the butter, scallion, rosemary, $1/2$ teaspoon of salt, pepper, lemon juice, and $1/4$ cup of the reserved cooking liquid. Hand mash until combined and the consistency you want, adding more cooking liquid if you wish.

Taste; you may want to add a pinch or two of sea salt. Serve hot.

VARIATION: For a richer mash, use Almond Milk (page 195) instead of the cooking liquid to thin the mash.

COOK'S NOTE: There's a good reason to use good old elbow grease when mashing starchy vegetables like potatoes. A food processor will turn them into a gluey mess.

PER SERVING: Calories: 170; Total Fat: 4 g (3 g saturated, 0 g mono-unsaturated); Carbohydrates: 30 g; Protein: 4 g; Fiber: 4 g; Sodium: 238 mg

STORAGE: Store in an airtight container in the refrigerator for up to 4 days.

1 pound rutabagas, peeled and cut into $1/2$-inch dice

Sea salt

Classic Magic Mineral Broth (page 44), Old-Fashioned Chicken Stock (page 46), store-bought organic stock, or water (room temperature)

$1^{1}/2$ pounds Yukon gold potatoes, peeled and cut into $1/2$-inch dice

2 tablespoons butter or ghee, or 3 tablespoons extra-virgin olive oil

1 large scallion, minced

$1/2$ teaspoon finely minced fresh rosemary

$1/4$ teaspoon freshly ground black pepper

$1/4$ teaspoon freshly squeezed lemon juice

Cauliflower Tabbouleh

MAKES 6 SERVINGS · PREP TIME: 15 minutes · COOK TIME: 20 minutes

Some foods just look like they should be good for the mind. Take cauliflower. Kind of like walnuts, it visually reminds you of the brain. And sure enough, cauliflower is a brain-boosting superstar, filled with B vitamins, omega-3s, phosphorus, and manganese. It helps in liver detoxification, and a happy liver—the body's vacuum cleaner for toxic metals—makes for a happy brain. Working with cauliflower can intimidate people—it's big and unwieldy—but it need not. In this tabbouleh, it goes incognito as what looks like rice or couscous, surrounded by spices, fresh green herbs, cucumber, and cherry tomatoes. It's a great dish for people who are watching their carbs but who want a grainlike taste and texture on which to munch.

1 1/2 pounds cauliflower, trimmed and cut into 1-inch florets

6 tablespoons freshly squeezed lemon juice

6 tablespoons extra-virgin olive oil

1/2 teaspoon ground turmeric

1/4 teaspoon ground coriander

1/4 teaspoon ground cumin

1/8 teaspoon ground cinnamon

Sea salt

1/4 teaspoon freshly ground pepper

1 cup tightly packed coarsely chopped parsley

1/2 cup coarsely chopped tightly packed mint

1/2 medium cucumber, peeled, seeded, and diced

12 cherry tomatoes, halved

Place the cauliflower florets in a steamer basket and steam until just tender-crisp, 5 to 6 minutes. Remove from the heat and let cool slightly. Place the cooked cauliflower in the bowl of a food processor and pulse about 15 times, until the texture is fine, with pieces about the size of rice grains.

In a large bowl whisk together lemon juice, olive oil, turmeric, coriander, cumin, cinnamon, 1/2 teaspoon of salt, and pepper. Add the cauliflower and toss well to coat. Taste, and adjust with a couple of pinches of salt if needed.

When the cauliflower has completely cooled, fold in the parsley, mint, cucumber, and tomatoes. Serve at room temperature.

COOK'S NOTE: If you thought cauliflower was just white, how about purple or cheddar orange for a change of pace? The new colors are the result of decades of traditional selective breeding to create more nutrient-dense food (this is not to be confused with, and has no relation to, genetically modified foods). Purple cauliflower has more brain-boosting anthocyanins, while the orange contains more beta-carotene. The best part—these glorious colors hold up even after cooking.

PER SERVING: Calories: 169; Total Fat: 15 g (2 g saturated, 11 g mono-unsaturated); Carbohydrates: 10 g; Protein: 3 g; Fiber: 4 g; Sodium: 178 mg

STORAGE: Store in an airtight container in the refrigerator for up to 3 days.

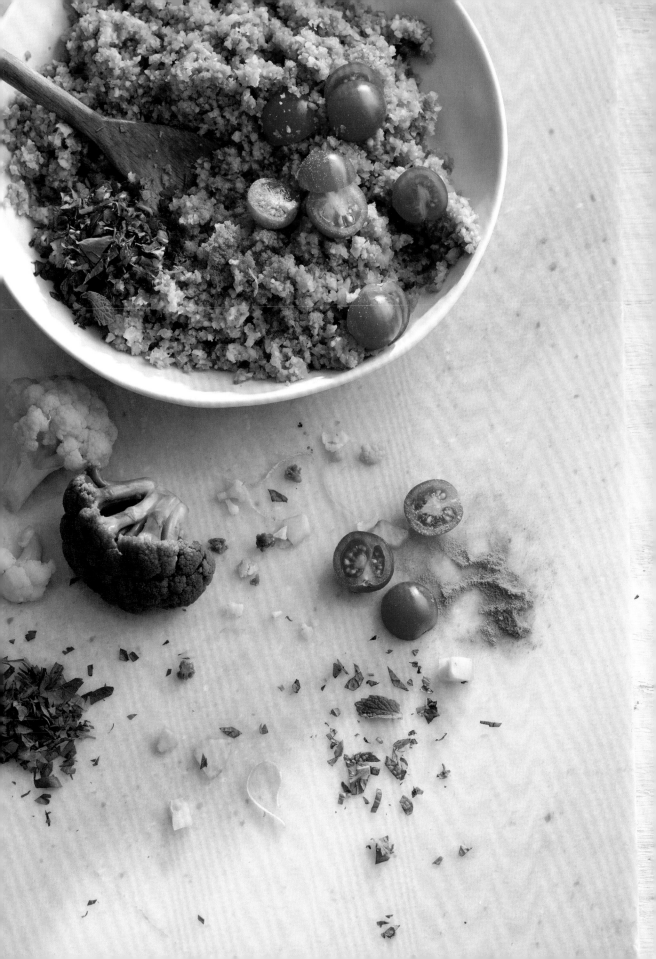

Riced Cauliflower Pilaf

MAKES 6 SERVINGS · PREP TIME: 15 minutes · COOK TIME: 20 minutes

And now, here's another magic trick to play with cauliflower, going from the macro to the micro. Pulsed into pieces the size of rice grains, the cauliflower carouses with other sautéed veggies—celery, carrots, and onions—and gains a golden halo from a hint of saffron. Saffron, which comes from the crocus plant, is one powerful brain spice, protecting the central nervous system from damage. It also contains serotonin precursors that may help improve mood. I know its taste certainly improves *my* mood.

$1/4$ heaping teaspoon saffron

3 tablespoons extra-virgin olive oil

3 small carrots, peeled and diced small

3 stalks celery, diced small

1 onion, diced small

Sea salt

$1^1/2$ pounds cauliflower, trimmed and cut into florets (about $4^1/2$ cups florets)

1 cup Old-Fashioned Chicken Stock (page 46), Classic Magic Mineral Broth (page 44), or store-bought organic stock

$1/8$ teaspoon freshly ground black pepper

2 teaspoons lemon zest

1 tablespoon freshly squeezed lemon juice

3 tablespoons chopped fresh parsley

In a small bowl, combine the saffron with 1 tablespoon of hot water; set aside.

Heat the olive oil in a large saucepan over medium heat, then add the carrots, celery, onions, and a pinch of salt and sauté for about 7 minutes, until the vegetables start to sweat and turn a golden color.

Meanwhile, place the cauliflower florets in the bowl of a food processor, in two batches if necessary. Pulse about 15 times, until the texture is small and resembles rice. Stir the cauliflower and saffron (with its water) into the pan with the sautéed vegetables, then stir in the stock, $1/4$ teaspoon of salt, and pepper and bring to a boil over high heat. Lower the heat to medium, cover, and simmer for about 8 minutes, until the cauliflower is tender.

Remove the pan's lid and cook until the broth has reduced, another 2 to 3 minutes. Remove from the heat and fluff with a fork, then add the lemon zest, lemon juice, and parsley and fluff again. Taste; you may want to add an additional pinch of salt.

Transfer to a serving bowl and serve immediately.

COOK'S NOTE: Turmeric is often considered the poor man's saffron, but it's no less of a super brain-boosting anti-inflammatory spice. It makes a great substitute when you don't have saffron.

PER SERVING: Calories: 78; Total Fat: 3 g (.5 g saturated, 2 g monounsaturated); Carbohydrates: 12.5 g; Protein: 3 g; Fiber: 4 g; Sodium: 142 mg

STORAGE: Store in an airtight container in the refrigerator for up to 3 days.

Castilian Cauliflower

MAKES 6 SERVINGS · PREP TIME: 15 minutes · COOK TIME: 20 minutes

Half the challenge of being a cook is staying out of a rut—that feeling that you're just cooking the "same old thing" again and again (it's like the culinary equivalent of the movie *Groundhog Day*). So it goes with cauliflower: it's such an important brain-boosting food, helping DNA function properly, and yet many people struggle with new ways to serve it up. If that's your issue, this recipe will help. Here we're using a food processor to pulse cauliflower into a ricelike state, and then plump it up by simmering it in chicken stock or vegetable broth. A hint of oregano, tomatoes, and olives is all it takes to morph this cauliflower from the mundane to the magnificent.

Heat the olive oil in a large skillet over medium heat, add the onion and a generous pinch of salt, and sauté until tender and slightly golden, about 7 minutes. Stir in the garlic, paprika, and chili powder and sauté another 30 seconds.

Meanwhile, place the cauliflower florets in the bowl of a food processor, in two batches if necessary. Pulse about 15 times, until the texture is small and resembles rice.

To the onion, add the cauliflower, 1/4 teaspoon of salt, pepper, broth, tomatoes, and oregano, stirring to combine. Bring to a simmer over medium-low heat, cover, and cook, stirring occasionally, until the cauliflower is tender, about 4 minutes. Remove the lid and continue cooking until the remaining liquid has evaporated and the cauliflower is completely tender, another 2 or 3 minutes. Stir in the lemon juice, maple syrup, and olives; taste and add another pinch of salt if needed.

Transfer to a serving bowl and serve immediately.

COOK'S NOTE: Chopping cauliflower releases enzymes that increase the bioavailability of its nutrients. Delaying the cooking for 5 to 10 minutes after cutting helps ensure the heat won't destroy the effectiveness of these enzymes. The enzymes also need vitamin C to activate, which is accomplished here with a hit of lemon juice.

PER SERVING: Calories: 164; Total Fat: 10.5 g (1.5 g saturated, 7 g monounsaturated); Carbohydrates: 15g; Protein: 3.5 g; Fiber: 4.5 g; Sodium: 394 mg

STORAGE: Store in an airtight container in the refrigerator for up to 2 days or in the freezer for up to 3 months.

3 tablespoons extra-virgin olive oil

1 small onion, diced small

Sea salt

2 tablespoons minced garlic

1 teaspoon paprika

1/2 teaspoon chili powder

1 1/2 pounds cauliflower, trimmed and cut into florets

1/4 teaspoon freshly ground black pepper

1 cup Classic Magic Mineral Broth (page 44), Old-Fashioned Chicken Stock (page 46), or store-bought organic stock

1 (15-ounce) can diced tomatoes

2 tablespoons minced fresh oregano

1 tablespoon freshly squeezed lemon juice

1/4 teaspoon Grade B maple syrup

3/4 cup pimento-stuffed olives, sliced

Ginger-Lime Sweet Potato Mash

MAKES 4 SERVINGS • PREP TIME: 5 minutes • COOK TIME 20 minutes

There's a fine line I walk as a cook. I don't want to take people too far out of their comfort zones, yet I want to energize their taste buds with delightful takes on old favorites. So it goes here. There are about 1,000 ways to prepare sweet potatoes, and mashing them is top of the list, but a simple twist takes these taters over the top, and that's the ginger (a notable anti-inflammatory) and the lime. Like a pair of piccolos, these two provide unexpected high notes of tartness and spice that play off the sweet potatoes' bass heartiness. If you're craving something sweet, this mash hits the mark; the fiber in the potatoes acts as a great insulin regulator, letting their sugars metabolize and feed the brain slowly and consistently.

$1^1/2$ pounds sweet potatoes or yams, peeled and cut into 2-inch cubes

Sea salt

Classic Magic Mineral Broth (page 44), Old-Fashioned Chicken Stock (page 46), store-bought organic stock, or water

2 tablespoons unsalted butter or ghee

1 tablespoon grated fresh ginger

$1/4$ teaspoon Grade B maple syrup

2 teaspoons freshly squeezed lime juice

1 tablespoon chopped fresh cilantro or mint, for garnish

Put the sweet potatoes and $1/4$ teaspoon of salt into a pot and add enough broth or other liquid to cover by 1 inch. Bring to a boil over high heat, then lower the heat to medium, cover, and simmer for 20 minutes, or until tender. Drain the potatoes in a colander, reserving the cooking water, and return them to the pot. Add the butter, ginger, maple syrup, $1/4$ teaspoon of salt, lime juice, and 2 to 3 tablespoons of the cooking liquid. Use a potato masher or electric hand mixer to mash the potatoes, adding more cooking liquid until you reach the desired consistency. Taste; you may want to add another pinch of salt or a squeeze of lime. Sprinkle with cilantro or mint and serve immediately.

VARIATIONS: Swap out the lime juice for orange juice and add a shaving of nutmeg. Garnish with mint or parsley rather than cilantro.

If you are avoiding dairy, substitute 2 tablespoons of extra-virgin olive oil or $1^1/2$ tablespoons of coconut oil for the 2 tablespoons of butter.

COOK'S NOTE: Here's a quick way to grate ginger. Cut the ginger so the yellow flesh is exposed, then run it across your Microplane. The ginger will collect on the underside, so give the grater a good tap and voilà—the ginger will release. You can also use this technique for grating garlic—just make sure to keep your fingertips from the grater edges.

PER SERVING: Calories: 199; Total Fat: 6 g (4 g saturated, 0 g mono-unsaturated); Carbohydrates: 35 g; Protein: 3 g; Fiber: 5 g; Sodium: 294 mg

Storage Time: Store in an airtight container in the refrigerator for 3 days.

Toasty Spiced Roasted Potatoes

MAKES 6 SERVINGS · PREP TIME: 10 minutes · COOK TIME: 30 minutes

Anybody who knows me knows I've got a potato jones that just won't quit. Doesn't matter the make and model, a properly prepared spud just takes me places. This version relies on a little spice razzamatazz: I throw some mustard and coriander seeds into a hot pan and play Jiffy Pop with them for about thirty seconds. It gets their oils going, and they get fully released—along with a load of anti-inflammatory ingredients—when I grind them a few seconds later. I then bake them along with some lovely fingerling potatoes coated with olive oil and sea salt, and it's heaven on a plate. Or so say the potato critics in my crowd, and they're not an easy bunch to please.

Preheat the oven to 450°F. Line a baking sheet with parchment paper.

Place a small pan over medium heat for a minute or two, until hot. Add the coriander and mustard seeds and swirl the pan over the heat for 30 to 60 seconds, until fragrant. Grind into a powder in a spice grinder or mortar and pestle. (See the Cook's Note.)

Put 2 tablespoons of the toasted spice mixture, olive oil, Dijon mustard, salt, and a few grinds of pepper in a large bowl and stir to combine. Add the potatoes and toss to evenly coat. Transfer the potatoes to the prepared baking sheet, spreading in a single layer. Bake, turning occasionally, for about 30 minutes, or until the potatoes begin to turn golden brown.

Transfer to a serving bowl and serve immediately.

COOK'S NOTE: This recipe makes three times the amount of ground coriander and mustard seeds you'll need; store the extra so you can roast these potatoes at a moment's notice. Store them in a jar for up to 3 months.

3 tablespoons coriander seeds

3 tablespoons mustard seeds

2 tablespoons extra-virgin olive oil

1 tablespoon plus 1 teaspoon Dijon mustard

1/2 teaspoon sea salt

Freshly ground black pepper

1 1/2 pounds fingerling potatoes, scrubbed and quartered lengthwise

PER SERVING: Calories: 158; Total Fat: 7 g (1 g saturated, 5 g monounsaturated); Carbohydrates: 23 g; Protein: 4 g; Fiber: 4.5 g; Sodium: 184 mg

STORAGE: Store in an airtight container in the refrigerator for up to 5 days.

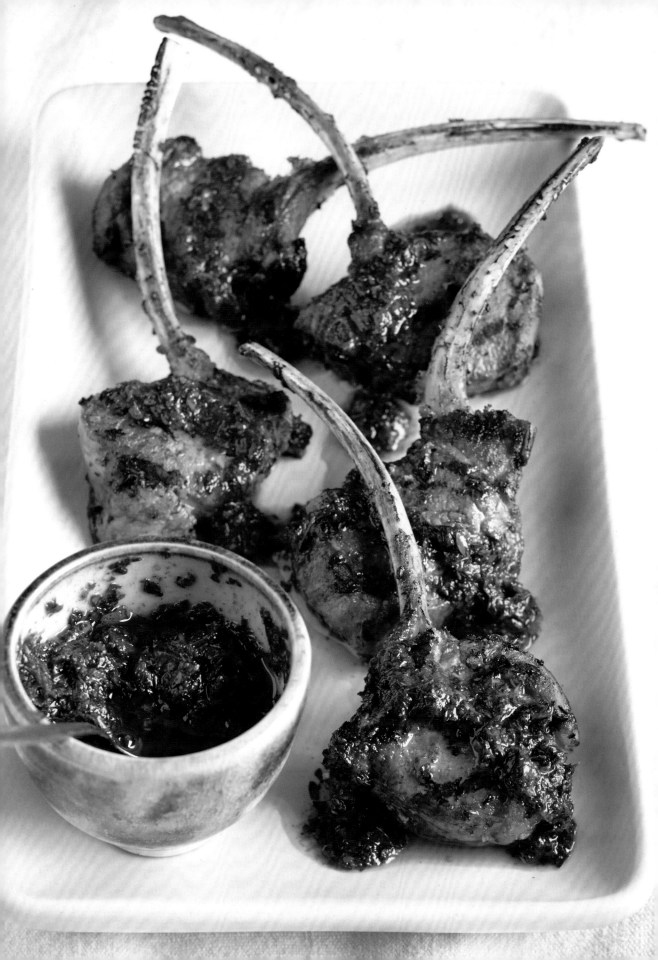

CHAPTER 6

Meat and Seafood

Though the brain is mostly made up of fat, it needs its proteins as well. Without foods like meat and seafood that contain proteins (and their precursors, amino acids), there would be no neurotransmitters, the chemicals that tell our brain what to do and when to do it. Dopamine (which signals reward and motivation), serotonin (emotion and impulses), glutamate (learning and memory): all are built from dietary sources of protiens. When shopping for meat and seafood, it's critical to buy the best quality you can find, including wild-caught (not farmed) fish and seafood, pasture-raised chicken, and grass-fed beef. There's a reason. Take beef: the nutritional profile of grass-fed beef is far superior to its feedlot-raised equivalent. Studies show it is far lower in cholesterol (22 percent versus 39 percent), higher in beta-carotene (perhaps twice as much), and full of good brain-healthy omega-3 fats. A single 4-ounce serving of grass-fed beef also contains more than half the daily recommended intake of protein and vitamin B12. Vitamin B12, which is mostly only found in meat and seafood (with the exceptions of flaxseed and nutritional yeast), is vital to a gene-control process known as methylation. Good methylation and the ability to metabolize B12 is absolutely necessary for keeping the body detoxified, repairing DNA, and for helping us avoid depression, irritability, and cognitive decline. Does grass-fed beef cost more? Yes, but the cost is offset by the fact that a little goes a long way. These recipes are so flavorful and nutrient-dense that the meat and seafood are just part of the dish, in contrast to the typical American plate, where the meat and seafood sit large and in charge. Once you see meat and seafood as important supporting players, rather than leads, you'll have a newfound appreciation for how they can be great flavor carriers for spices and herbs, which are also keys to a healthier, happier brain.

Shrimp-Stuffed Avocados 2.0

MAKES 4 SERVINGS · PREP TIME: 10 minutes · COOK TIME: 4 minutes

As a kid, I remember the Ladies Who Lunch coming over to the house regularly to play canasta or mah-jongg. On these occasions, my mom showed me how you could use a fruit as a bowl for salad: she'd serve the pearled grand dames tomatoes stuffed with chicken salad, and that was the inspiration for this dish. I've gone for a different mode of transport—an avocado boat—and jazzed up the salad as well. No mayo here, but lime juice, cumin, coriander, jalapeño (za-zing!), olive oil, and avocado provide the diving pond for the shrimp. I think the Ladies Who Lunch would've approved.

DRESSING

1/2 cup coarsely chopped cilantro

1/4 cup coarsely chopped parsley

1/4 cup extra-virgin olive oil

3 tablespoons freshly squeezed lime juice

1/2 teaspoon ground cumin

1/4 teaspoon ground coriander

1 jalapeño, seeded and chopped

1 clove garlic, peeled and smashed

1/4 teaspoon sea salt

2 large ripe avocados

Freshly squeezed lemon or lime juice

Sea salt

1 pound cooked shrimp, cut into bite-size pieces

1 Granny Smith apple, cut into bite-size pieces

2 scallions, sliced

1 tablespoon pumpkin seeds, toasted (optional)

To make the dressing, combine the cilantro, parsley, olive oil, lime juice, cumin, coriander, jalapeño, garlic, and salt in a food processor and process until smooth.

Cut the avocados in half and remove the pits. Spritz the cut flesh with lemon or lime juice and sprinkle with salt. Make a well in the avocado halves by scooping out some, of the flesh, leaving a 1/2-inch border. Place the flesh in a bowl and mash it lightly with a fork. Add the shrimp, apple, and scallion and 4 tablespoons of the dressing; stir until evenly coated. (Reserve the rest of the dressing for another use; it will keep for 5 days in the fridge.)

Spoon the shrimp mixture into the well of the avocado halves, making a nice mounded scoop in each. Sprinkle with toasted pumpkin seeds and serve immediately.

PER SERVING: Calories: 436; Total Fat: 31 g (4 g saturated, 21 g mono-unsaturated); Carbohydrates: 12.5 g; Protein: 31 g; Fiber: 8 g; Sodium: 435 mg

STORAGE: The shrimp salad, sans avocado, will store in an airtight container in the refrigerator for up to 2 days. The dressing will store in an airtight container in the refrigerator for up to 5 days.

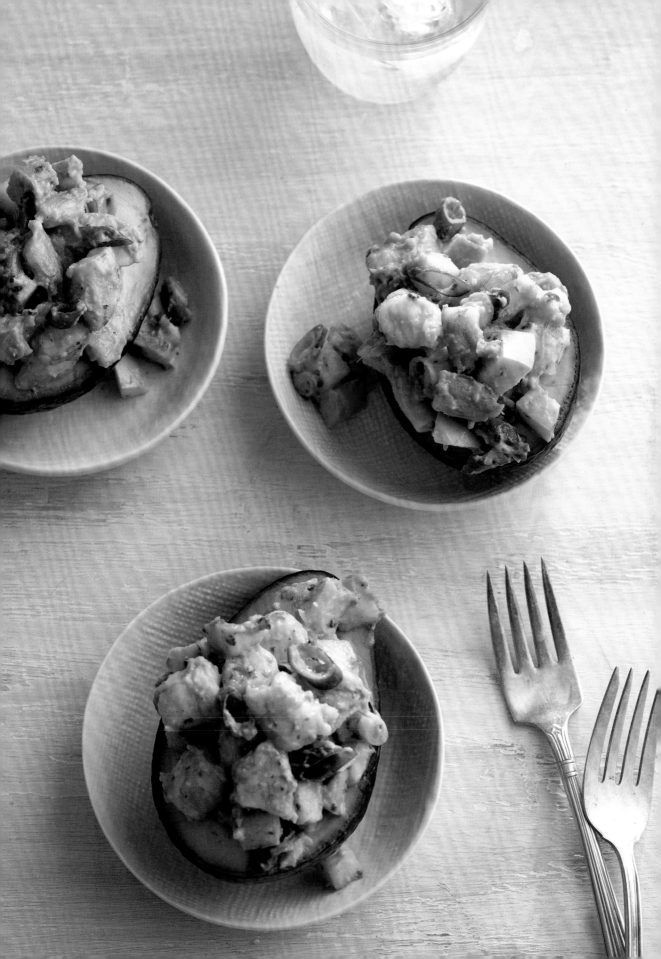

Simple Shrimp Scampi

MAKES 4 SERVINGS • PREP TIME: 10 minutes • COOK TIME: 10 minutes

A lot of people think "simple" and "scampi" couldn't possibly go together, but I'm here to say that isn't the case. Scampi is simply an Italian style of cooking a big mama of a shrimp doused with olive oil, garlic, and a splash of white wine. That's pretty simple in my book. The only thing you really need to do is keep a sharp eye on the stove, because once the garlic hits the pan it cooks mighty fast (as do the shrimp; 3 minutes is all it takes). As a brain booster, shrimp's B12 can't be beat, and the anti-inflammatory benefits of garlic are superb.

2 tablespoons extra-virgin olive oil

3 teaspoons minced garlic

1/4 teaspoon red pepper flakes

1/2 cup dry white wine

1 pound large shrimp, peeled and deveined

Sea salt

2 teaspoons lemon zest

Freshly squeezed lemon juice

2 tablespoons finely chopped fresh parsley

Heat the olive oil in a heavy skillet over medium heat. Add the garlic and red pepper flakes and sauté for 30 seconds, until the garlic is fragrant and slightly golden. Add 1/4 cup of the wine and deglaze the pan, scraping up any bits that are stuck to the pan, and cook until the liquid has reduced by half. Add the shrimp, a pinch of salt, and the remaining wine. Cook until the shrimp is opaque, about 3 minutes. Gently stir in the lemon zest, 2 teaspoons of lemon juice, and parsley. Taste; you may want to add another pinch of salt and a squeeze of lemon juice. Serve immediately.

PER SERVING: Calories: 178; Total Fat: 8.5 g (1 g saturated, 6 g mono-unsaturated); Carbohydrates: 3 g; Protein: 16 g; Fiber: 0 g; Sodium: 693 mg

STORAGE: Store in an airtight container in the fridge for 2 days.

Curried Shrimp

WITH JAPANESE SWEET POTATO

MAKES 4 SERVINGS • PREP TIME: 15 minutes • COOK TIME: 30 minutes

Curry is one of those dishes that conjures up an image of a sous chef flying between four pans at once, flames leaping, cooks yelling. But this curry takes place all in one pan, all the elements cooked sequentially: first the spices, then the broth, and finally the shrimp. This is definitely the kind of dish you'd order in a Thai restaurant and wonder, "How can it come out so fast?" Answer: they have their broth ready to go; it's just a matter of adding the rest of the ingredients. Here the rest of our ingredients are a load of goodness: turmeric, ginger, basil, sweet potatoes, red bell peppers, cauliflower, sweet potatoes, and, of course, omega-3-rich shrimp. This is mental health in a pan. (Just one.)

Heat the coconut oil over medium-low heat. Add the curry paste and turmeric, mix, and spread around the pan. Stir in the ginger, then the onion and a pinch of salt and sauté about 3 minutes. Add 1/4 cup of the broth, stirring to remove any bits stuck to the pot, and cook until the liquid is reduced by half. Add the sweet potato and toss to coat. Add the coconut milk and the remainder of the broth, fish sauce, and kaffir lime leaves. Bring to a simmer, then decrease the heat. Cover and cook until the sweet potato is just tender, about 10 minutes.

Stir in the bell pepper, cauliflower, and string beans and simmer, covered, until crisp-tender, about 8 minutes. Gently stir in the shrimp and simmer until cooked through and just opaque, about 4 minutes. Add the lime juice, and taste; you may want to add a bit of salt and another squeeze of lime juice. Remove the kaffir lime leaves.

Transfer to a serving dish, garnish with the Thai basil and cilantro, and serve immediately.

COOK'S NOTE: A Japanese sweet potato is white-fleshed and has a firmer texture when cooked. It's also not as sweet as its orange cousin. If you can't find one, use a regular sweet potato.

PER SERVING: Calories: 403; Total Fat: 26 g (21.5 g saturated, 1 g monounsaturated); Carbohydrates: 27 g; Protein: 21.5 g; Fiber: 5 g; Sodium: 900 mg (sodium from the shrimp, fish sauce, and red curry paste)

STORAGE: Store in an airtight container in the refrigerator for up to 3 days.

1 tablespoon coconut oil or other neutral oil, such as grapeseed oil

1 tablespoon red curry paste

1 teaspoon ground turmeric

1 tablespoon minced fresh ginger

1 yellow onion, cut in 1/2-inch dice

Sea salt

1/2 cup Classic Magic Mineral Broth (page 44) or store-bought organic stock

8 ounces Japanese or white flesh sweet potato, peeled, quartered, and cut into 1/2-inch slices

1 (13 1/2 ounce) can unsweetened coconut milk

1 tablespoon fish sauce

2 kaffir lime leaves, or 1 teaspoon lime zest

1 cup 1/2-inch-diced red bell pepper

1 cup cauliflower florets

1 cup 1-inch-sliced string beans

1 pound large shrimp, peeled and deveined

1 teaspoon freshly squeezed lime juice

2 tablespoons chopped Thai basil leaves or mint, for garnish

2 tablespoons chopped cilantro, for garnish

Pan-Seared Curried Scallops

MAKES 4 SERVINGS · PREP TIME: 5 minutes · COOK TIME: 6 minutes

Scallops are an awesome brain food, full of the omega-3 fatty acid called DHA, which reduces plaque formations in the brain linked to cognitive decline. However, they're a bit temperamental on the stove. They cook mighty fast, and can turn from tender to eraser-tough in a flash. Pay attention, and you'll get a plateful of bliss. Here, they're seasoned with curry and a little coconut and lime, which play beautifully off the scallops' silky taste. Serve these with Ginger Scented Forbidden Rice (page 143), Ginger-Lime Sweet Potato Mash (page 100), or Coconut Ginger Lime Kale (page 86).

12 dry-packed sea scallops

Sea salt

1 teaspoon curry powder

2 tablespoons extra-virgin olive oil, butter, ghee or coconut oil

2 teaspoons grated fresh ginger

1 cup coconut milk

1 tablespoon freshly squeezed lime juice

1 teaspoon snipped fresh chives, or 1 minced scallion, for garnish

Rinse the scallops, then pat very dry with paper towels. This step is very important, especially if you're using frozen scallops; if they aren't dry, you'll be steaming instead of searing them. Season both sides of the scallops with salt and sprinkle the curry powder over both sides of the scallops. Give each one a pat so the curry becomes evenly distributed over the surface.

Heat the olive oil in a large skillet over medium-high heat, then add the scallops to the pan one at a time in a single uncrowded layer. Cook them in two batches if necessary. Let cook undisturbed, until deep golden-brown on the bottom, about 2 minutes. Turn and sear the other side until golden and the internal temperature registers between 150°F and 155°F, another 2 minutes. The scallops should be almost firm to the touch. Transfer the scallops to a serving plate and keep warm.

Turn the heat down to medium-low and add the grated ginger to the pan. Cook until fragrant, about 30 seconds. Stir in the coconut milk to deglaze the skillet, scraping any loose bits stuck to the pan. Cook the sauce until slightly thickened, about 1 minute. Stir in the lime juice and any accumulated juices from the scallops. Taste; you might want to add a pinch or two of salt. Spoon the coconut sauce over the scallops, garnish with the chives, and serve immediately.

PER SERVING: Calories: 191 Total Fat: 17 g (4 g saturated, 11 g mono-unsaturated); Carbohydrates: 5 g; Protein: 6 g; Fiber: 0.5 g; Sodium: 465 mg

STORAGE: Store in an airtight container in the refrigerator for up to 2 days.

Baked Halibut

WITH TOMATO, MINT, AND FENNEL VINAIGRETTE

MAKES 4 SERVINGS · PREP TIME: 5 minutes plus 20 minutes to marinate · COOK TIME: 10 to 12 minutes

Halibut is a very forgiving fish; you can top it with just about anything and it'll taste great. Many of the dollops (pages 163 to 185) work well, but I especially like the Tomato, Mint, and Fennel Vinaigrette (page 173). It's not just the flashy look (although it certainly is eye-catching), but also the big, bold flavor, which includes fennel, Dijon mustard, and kalamata olives.

Combine the lemon juice, lemon zest, oregano, salt, and olive oil in a small bowl and whisk until thoroughly blended. Spread the marinade over both sides of the fish fillets. Cover and refrigerate for 20 minutes.

Preheat the oven to 400°F. Lightly oil an ovenproof pan large enough to accommodate all of the fillets in a single layer.

Drain the fillets, discarding the marinade, and pat them dry with paper towels. Put the fish in the prepared pan and bake for 10 to 12 minutes, until the flesh is opaque and flakes easily. To be certain the fish is cooked through, push a two-pronged kitchen fork straight down into the flesh; the fish is done when it is no longer translucent at the center of the thickest part of the fillet.

Top each fillet with the Tomato, Mint, and Fennel Vinaigrette and serve immediately.

COOK'S NOTES: Instead of baking, you can grill the halibut. Marinate as directed, then wipe off the marinade. Rub 1/4 teaspoon of grapeseed oil over each fillet, then grill over low, even heat for about 4 minutes per side, until the flesh is opaque and flakes easily and the center of each fillet registers 135°F.

It's best to buy fillets of halibut cut from smaller fish (twenty pounds and under). These fish are younger and have the highest levels of omega-3s. Usually, it's best to buy your fish the same day you're preparing it. If you must store the fish longer, put it in a resealable plastic bag in the coldest part of your refrigerator, usually the back of the bottom shelf. It should hold for an extra two days.

PER SERVING: Calories: 287 Total Fat: 14 g (2.5 g saturated, 9 g mono-unsaturated); Carbohydrates: 5.5 g; Protein: 35 g; Fiber: 1 g; Sodium: 369 mg

STORAGE: Store in an airtight container in the refrigerator for up to 2 days.

4 (6-ounce) halibut fillets

2 tablespoons freshly squeezed lemon juice

1 teaspoon grated lemon zest

1 tablespoon fresh oregano, chopped, or 1/4 teaspoon dried oregano

1/4 teaspoon sea salt

2 tablespoons extra-virgin olive oil

1/2 cup Tomato, Mint, and Fennel Vinaigrette (page 173)

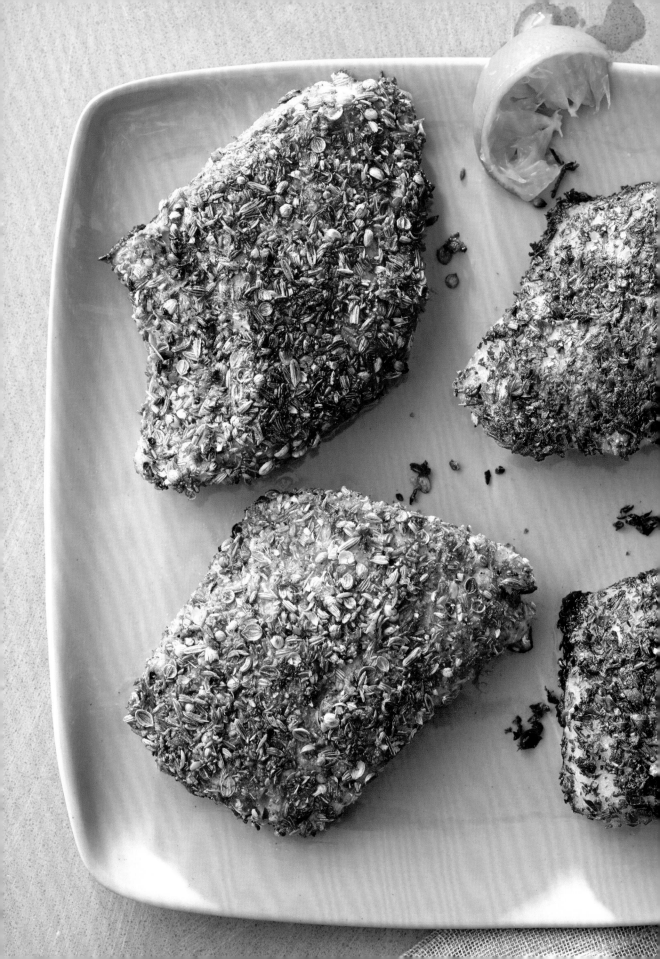

Black Cod Duvet

MAKES 4 SERVINGS • PREP TIME: 10 minutes plus 30 minutes for seasoning • COOK TIME: 10 minutes

What do a fish in a kitchen and a human at a spa have in common? Tight, snuggly blankets. Follow me here: spas use mylar blankets to wrap up people who've gotten mineral treatments so the nutrients will sink deep into their pores. Similarly, cooks wrap fish to make sure herbs or spices sink deeply into the flesh. Just choose your preferred crust, pat the herbs or spices on the fish, wrap it snug, and 30 minutes later you've got an amazingly seasoned fillet ready to cook. Black cod (aka sablefish) is a great brain booster, with the richest omega-3 profile of any fish in the sea.

Pat the fish dry and portion into 4 pieces. Season both sides of each piece with salt and pepper, and set aside while you make the herb or spice crust.

To make the herb-crusted fish: In a baking dish or on a large plate, mix together the salt, pepper, parsley, oregano, thyme, and sage. Place the fish on the herbs and pat them firmly onto both sides.

To make the spice-crusted fish: Coarsely grind the salt, pepper, cumin, coriander, fennel seeds, and red pepper flakes in a spice grinder and place in a small bowl. Spread the top of each piece evenly with 1 teaspoon of Dijon mustard, then sprinkle with one-fourth of the spice mixture, gently patting to create an even crust on one side.

Place the herbed or spiced fish on sheets of plastic wrap, patting any leftover herbs or spices into the top. Wrap the fish pieces snugly and put them in the fridge for at least 30 minutes or up to overnight to infuse the flavors and help the crust adhere.

Preheat the oven to 400°F.

Over medium-high heat, heat the olive oil in an oven-safe skillet large enough to hold all the fish without crowding. When the oil is hot, place the fish in the pan (crust side down if you're using the spice crust) and cook for 3 minutes. Flip the fish over and place the pan in the oven for another 3 to 4 minutes to finish cooking, until the flesh is opaque and flakes easily. Serve immediately.

PER SERVING (Herb Crust): Calories: 142; Total Fat: 8 g (1 g saturated, 6 g monounsaturated); Carbohydrates: 1 g; Protein: 17.5 g; Fiber: 0 g; Sodium: 396 mg

PER SERVING (Spice Crust): Calories: 147; Total Fat: 8 g (1 g saturated, 6 g monounsaturated); Carbohydrates: 1.5 g; Protein: 18 g; Fiber: 1 g; Sodium: 461 mg

STORAGE: Store in an airtight container in the refrigerator for up to 2 days.

1 pound black cod or halibut fillets

Sea salt

Freshly ground black pepper

HERB CRUST

1/4 teaspoon sea salt

1/8 teaspoon freshly ground black pepper

1/4 cup finely chopped parsley

1 tablespoon finely chopped fresh oregano

2 teaspoons finely chopped fresh thyme

2 teaspoons finely chopped fresh sage

SPICE CRUST

1/4 teaspoon sea salt

1/8 teaspoon freshly ground black pepper

4 teaspoons Dijon mustard

2 teaspoons cumin seed

2 teaspoons coriander seed

1 teaspoon fennel seed

Pinch of red pepper flakes

2 tablespoons extra-virgin olive oil

Wild Salmon Kebabs
WITH ASIAN PESTO

MAKES 4 SERVINGS • PREP TIME: 10 minutes plus 30 minutes to marinate • COOK TIME: Less than 10 minutes

Sometimes it's just fun to play with your food. I want people to eat omega-3 rich wild salmon—it's great for heart and brain health—and this recipe is a blast. The salmon is cubed, threaded onto skewers, baked for a few minutes, and voilà: instant salmon kebabs. The Asian pesto, with ginger, cilantro, and mint, makes the skewers a kick to eat. I like this dish served with Watercress, Purple Cabbage, and Edamame Salad with Toasted Sesame Seeds (page 75). Talk about a color blast!

ASIAN PESTO

1 tablespoon minced ginger

1 clove garlic, minced

1 scallion, chopped

1 tablespoon finely chopped seeded jalapeño

3/4 cup tightly packed cilantro leaves

1/4 cup tightly packed fresh mint leaves

1/4 cup tightly packed flat-leaf parsley

3 tablespoons extra-virgin olive oil

1/4 teaspoon sea salt

2 tablespoons freshly squeezed lime juice

1/4 teaspoon Grade B maple syrup

1 pound wild salmon fillet, skin and pinbones removed

Sea salt

Freshly ground black pepper

Line a rimmed baking sheet with parchment paper and set aside. Place bamboo skewers in a bowl of water for a few minutes, until soaked through.

To make the Asian pesto, put the ginger, garlic, scallion, jalapeño, cilantro, mint, parsley, oil, salt, lime juice, and maple syrup into a small food processor. Blend until smooth, about a minute.

Place the salmon on a cutting board and cut it lengthwise, then crosswise into 8 equal pieces. Put the fish on the prepared baking sheet. Insert a 6-inch bamboo skewer into each block of salmon so it looks like a rectangular lollipop. Sprinkle a bit of salt and pepper over each piece. Using half the pesto, spread it on all sides of each piece of salmon. Cover and refrigerate for 30 minutes.

Preheat the oven to 400°F.

Remove the salmon from the refrigerator, uncover, and slide the baking sheet into the oven. Bake just until an instant-read thermometer inserted into the center of the salmon registers 120°F, 7 to 9 minutes depending on the thickness of the fillets. The flesh should be just opaque and beginning to flake.

Transfer the kabobs, skewers and all, to a serving plate. Add a dollop of the remaining pesto to each piece of salmon and serve immediately.

COOK'S NOTES: To get pieces that are of even thickness, purchase the center cut of the salmon rather than the tail.

Cut the baked salmon up into smaller pieces and stick in toothpicks. Serve with the additional pesto on the side for great little appetizers.

PER SERVING: Calories: 266; Total Fat: 17 g (3 g saturated, 11 g monounsaturated); Carbohydrates: 2.5 g; Protein: 25 g; Fiber: 1 g; Sodium: 157 mg

STORAGE: Store in an airtight container in the refrigerator for up to 2 days.

Mediterranean Sockeye Salmon Salad

MAKES 2 SERVINGS · PREP TIME: 10 minutes · COOK TIME: Not applicable

I'm a realist when it comes to fish. Sometimes the urge hits, but a) you don't want to run down to the market and, b) you don't feel like cooking up a salmon steak. That's why canned salmon was invented, but it can get boring if all you do is smush it around with some mayonnaise. So here's my answer, a different way of approaching a quick salmon hit. I take it to the Mediterranean, where chopped kalamata olives, capers, parsley, olive oil, and a bit of Dijon mustard put the salmon through its paces. The combination of the healthy monounsaturated fats from the olives and the nice dose of healthy omega-3s from the salmon provides healthy fat for the brain.

Put the salmon in a bowl and break it into small pieces with a fork.

Stir in the mustard, olives, 1 tablespoon of lemon juice, 1 tablespoon of olive oil, and a pinch of sea salt, the celery, red onion, capers, and parsley. Divide the arugula between 2 serving plates and drizzle with a little bit of lemon juice and olive oil and another pinch of salt. Spoon over the salmon salad and serve.

PER SERVING: Calories, 176; Total Fat 10 g (2 g saturated, 3 g monounsaturated); Carbohydrates: 2 g; Protein: 20 g; Fiber: 3 g; Sodium: 644 mg

STORAGE: Store refrigerated in an airtight container for 3 days.

1 (6-ounce) can sockeye salmon, drained

2 teaspoons Dijon mustard

12 kalamata olives, rinsed and coarsely chopped

Freshly squeezed lemon juice

Extra-virgin olive oil

Sea salt

2 tablespoons finely diced celery

2 teaspoons finely diced red onion

2 teaspoons capers, rinsed

2 tablespoons finely diced parsley

1/8 teaspoon freshly ground black pepper

3 cups arugula, rinsed and dried

Roasted Ginger Salmon
WITH POMEGRANATE OLIVE MINT SALSA

MAKES 4 SERVINGS · PREP TIME: 10 minutes plus 20 minutes to marinate · COOK TIME: 15 minutes

All I can say is get out your camera, cause when you make this dish, you're going to want to take a picture of it before you serve it. It's just that pretty, with the peach of the salmon, the ruby red jewels of the pomegranate seeds, the vibrant green of the parsley. The taste is no less sensational, the citrus and herbs playing wonderfully off the salmon's healthy blend of omega-3 rich fats. This one will energize all your senses.

1/2 cup freshly squeezed orange juice

2 tablespoons freshly squeezed lime juice

2 tablespoons freshly squeezed lemon juice

Zest of 1 orange

Zest of 1 lemon

1 tablespoon extra-virgin olive oil

1/2 teaspoon finely minced fresh ginger

Pinch of cayenne pepper

4 (6-ounce) salmon fillets, pinbones removed

Sea salt

1 teaspoon Dijon mustard

1 cup Pomegranate Olive Mint Salsa (page 182)

In a small bowl or glass measuring cup, whisk together the orange juice, lime juice, lemon juice, orange zest, lemon zest, olive oil, ginger, and cayenne. Place the salmon in a baking dish and season each piece with a pinch of salt. Pour half of the marinade over the salmon and turn to coat well. Cover the baking dish and marinate in the refrigerator for 20 minutes.

Preheat the oven to 400°F.

Remove the salmon from the refrigerator, uncover, and add 2 tablespoons of water to the dish. Bake for 10 to 15 minutes, depending on the thickness of the fillets, just until tender and opaque and an instant-read thermometer inserted into the center of the fillet registers 120°F.

While the salmon is cooking, combine the reserved marinade and the mustard in a small saucepan over medium heat and simmer until the liquid is reduced by half. Pour the reduction over the fillets. Spoon 1/4 cup of the relish on top of each fillet, and serve immediately.

COOK'S NOTE: Like Goldilocks and the three bears, fish has to be just right. Too much time in the oven or on the grill leaves your fish too dry. Too little time and you will have raw fish. As with many other proteins, fish continues to cook for several minutes after you take it off the heat. This is called carryover cooking. Let an instant-read thermometer be your guide and pull your fish away from the heat at 120°F. By the time you're ready to serve it, your fish will be perfect.

PER SERVING: Calories: 298 Total Fat: 14 g (3 g saturated, 6.5 g mono-unsaturated); Carbohydrates: 5 g; Protein: 37 g; Fiber: 0.5 g; Sodium: 195 mg

STORAGE: Store in an airtight container in the refrigerator for up to 3 days.

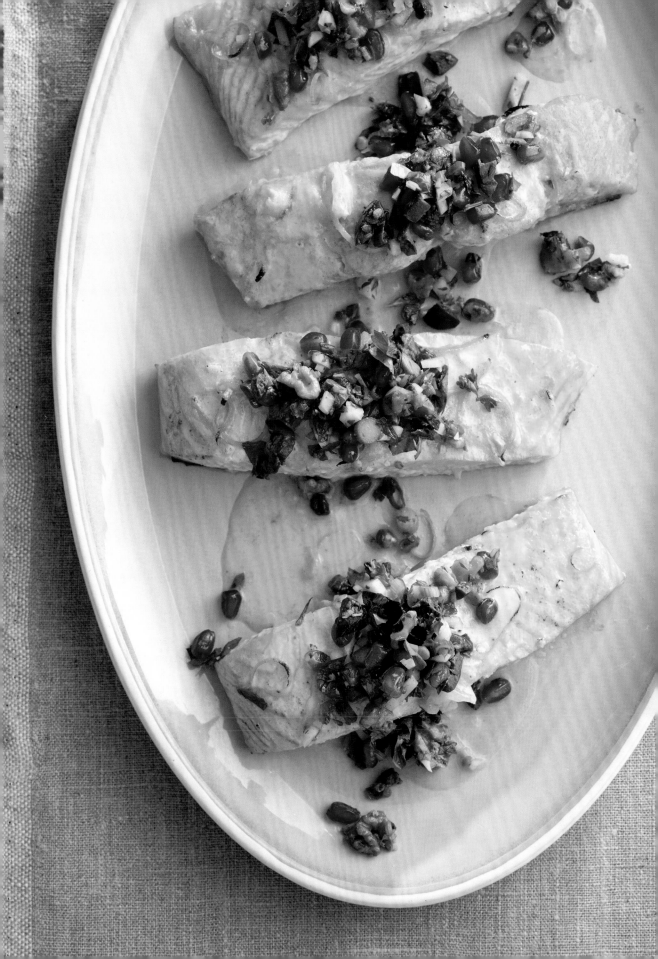

Quinoa Turkey Meatballs

Remember the famous episode of *I Love Lucy,* where Lucy slowly gets overwhelmed by the chocolate factory assembly line? Everything starts out fine, but before you know it she's stuffing chocolates into her mouth just to keep up. Making meatballs can feel that way—hand-rolling them gets stultifying mighty quickly. Here, you let the soup take the place of your hands; once the soup gets to a gentle boil, use a melon baller or tablespoon to form the meatballs and plop them into the broth. The broth does all the work, poaching each meatball to a perfect, fluffy roundness. You can also bake the meatballs and serve them with a sauce—like Roasted Tomato Sauce (page 167), or Signora Francini's Salsa Verde (page 174)—or with vegetables.

And what's in it for your brain health? In addition to the eggs in the meatball mixture providing a great source of choline (for healthy brain function), the turkey provides a nice relaxant in tryptophan.

1 large organic egg

1/2 cup scallions, thinly sliced

2 teaspoons minced garlic

1 teaspoon fennel seed

1 teaspoon lemon zest

1 1/2 tablespoons freshly chopped oregano or 1/2 teaspoon dried oregano

2 tablespoons finely chopped parsley

1/2 teaspoon sea salt

1/2 teaspoon freshly ground black pepper

1/2 cup cooked quinoa

12 ounces ground turkey

4 cups Old-Fashioned Chicken Stock (page 46), Italian Wedding Soup (page 66), or store-bought stock (optional, see Cook's Note)

To make the meatballs, whisk the egg in a bowl. Whisk in the scallions, garlic, fennel seed, lemon zest, oregano, parsley, salt, and pepper. Add the cooked quinoa and stir to combine. Add the turkey, and mix with your hands or a spatula until just combined (see Cook's Note).

Use a melon baller or tablespoon to scoop out balls of the turkey mixture, and either poach, bake, or freeze the meatballs. To poach, see the Cook's Note. To bake, evenly space the meatballs on a parchment-lined baking sheet, slip into a 400°F oven, and bake for 20 minutes. To freeze, evenly space the meatballs on a parchment-lined baking sheet and put in the freezer for about 30 minutes to 1 hour, until they're solid. Then transfer to a freezer bag or airtight container; the meatballs will and keep for up to 2 months. They can go straight from the freezer into a soup (simmer for about 12 minutes to poach), or bake for about 30 minutes at 400°F.

VARIATION: Substitute ground dark-meat chicken or grass-fed beef for the turkey meat.

COOK'S NOTE: Poach the meatballs in the Italian Wedding Soup (page 66) or any broth. The liquid should be just below the boiling point, with its surface barely quivering. Be careful not to overcrowd the pot, and work in batches so you can keep the cooking temperature up.

PER SERVING: Calories: 116; Total Fat: 5 g (1 g saturated, 1.5 g monounsaturated); Carbohydrates: 6 g; Protein: 11 g; Fiber: 2 g; Sodium: 149 mg

STORAGE: Store cooked meatballs in an airtight container in the refrigerator for up to 3 days.

Big Cat's Turkey Meatloaf
WITH NOT-SO-SECRET SAUCE

MAKES 6 SERVINGS · PREP TIME: 20 Minutes · COOK TIME: 1 hour

Tell some people *every* ingredient in a dish and they'll never try it. But if you wait until after they've tasted a to go into full disclosure, they'll be pleasantly stunned at what they've just eaten. This gluten-free meatloaf is kept moist by mushrooms—the idea of my cooking buddy Catherine McConkie—and has great umami flavor from anchovies. Just wait until they've tried it to tell your guests.

To make the sauce, heat the olive oil in a saucepan over medium-high heat. Add the onion and a pinch of salt. Sauté until translucent, 3 minutes, and add the garlic. Sauté about 30 seconds more, then stir in the tomato puree, syrup, vinegar, cinnamon, and salt. Reduce the heat to medium low, and simmer until thickened and reduced, stirring occasionally, about 40 minutes. Remove the cinnamon stick and set aside 1 cup of the sauce for the meatloaf (reserve the rest of the sauce for another use).

While the sauce is simmering, make the meatloaf. Preheat the oven to 350°F. Put the mushrooms in the bowl of a food processor and pulse until they are finely ground. Set aside.

Heat the olive oil in a medium skillet over medium heat. Add the onion and carrot and sauté until tender and golden, about 5 minutes. Add the red pepper flakes, garlic, anchovies, salt, and pepper, and sauté 1 minute more. Transfer the mixture to a bowl and stir in the mustard, oregano, thyme, parsley, and mushrooms, and mix to combine. Add turkey and mix gently with your hands, just to combine. Shape the meat to fit into an ovenproof dish. Top with the reserved 1 cup of sauce. Bake for 1 hour. Remove from the oven and allow the turkey meatloaf to rest, covered with aluminum foil, for 10 minutes. Slice and serve immediately.

PER SERVING: Calories: 192; Total Fat: 9.5 g (2 g saturated, 5 g mono-unsaturated); Carbohydrates: 5 g; Protein: 20 g; Fiber: 1 g; Sodium: 251 mg

STORAGE: Store in the refrigerator in an airtight container for up to 4 days. Freeze in an airtight container for 1 month.

SAUCE

2 tablespoons extra-virgin olive oil

1/2 cup small dice yellow onion

Sea salt

1 large clove garlic, minced

2 cups tomato puree

1/4 cup Grade B maple syrup

2 tablespoons apple cider vinegar

1 cinnamon stick

MEATLOAF

5 ounces cremini mushrooms, cleaned, trimmed, and sliced

2 tablespoons extra-virgin olive oil

1/2 yellow onion, diced small

1 small carrot, peeled and diced small

1/4 teaspoon red pepper flakes

2 tablespoons minced garlic

2 skinless, boneless anchovies, rinsed, and minced

1/2 teaspoon sea salt

1/4 teaspoon freshly ground black pepper

1 tablespoon Dijon mustard

1 1/2 tablespoons minced fresh oregano, or 2 teaspoons dried

1 tablespoon minced fresh thyme, or 1 1/2 teaspoons dried

1/2 cup chopped parsley

1 1/4 pounds ground turkey thigh meat

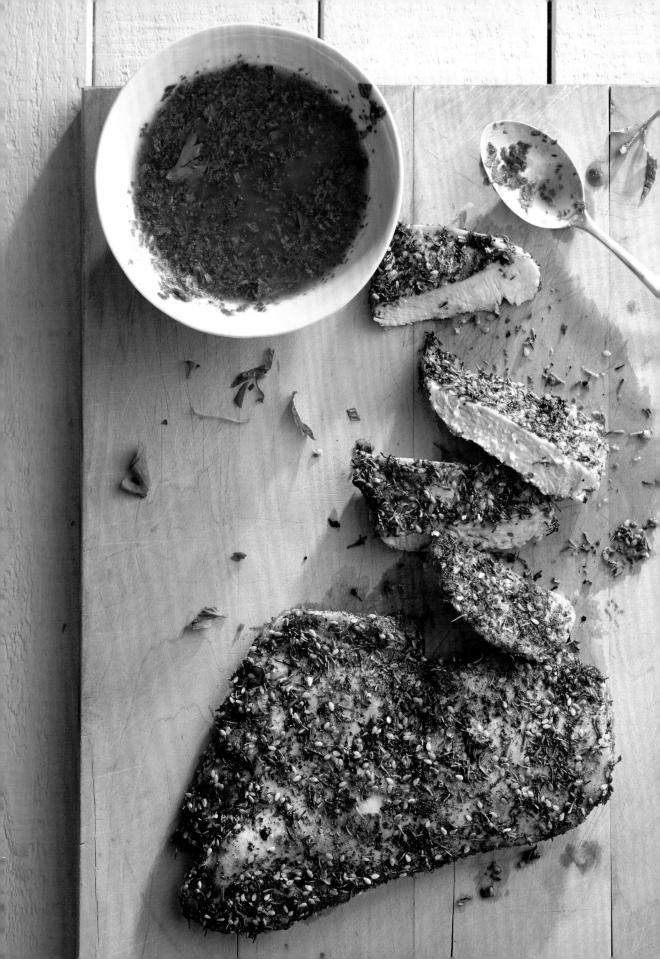

Grilled Chicken with Za'atar

MAKES 4 SERVINGS • PREP TIME: 15 minutes plus 30 minutes to marinate • COOK TIME: 5 minutes

Can you say "za'atar?" Sure you can. In fact, if you lived in the Middle East, you'd be invoking the name of this herb-and-spice mix nearly every day. *Za'atar* has long had a reputation as a brain enhancer, and science may be providing a clue; researchers wrote that, in low concentrations, the carvacrol found in oregano and thyme may increase feelings of well-being. Chicken is particularly rich in brain-enhancing nutrients. This recipe makes about half a cup of *za'atar*, which is a lot more than you need for the chicken; store the extra in a jar and use to sprinkle on top of vegetables, dips, salad dressings, fish, eggs, or anything you would like to add a touch of the exotic.

To make the *za'atar,* combine all the ingredients and mix well. Set aside 1 tablespoon to season the chicken and reserve the remainder for other uses.

To make the chicken, put the olive oil, *za'atar*, lemon zest, salt, and pepper in a small bowl and whisk until well blended.

Working with one piece at a time, put the chicken between several layers of parchment paper and pound with a meat pounder until about 1/4 inch thick. Put the chicken in a pan in which the pieces fit without overlapping. Spread the reserved tablespoon of *za'atar* evenly over the chicken, cover, and refrigerate for 15 to 30 minutes. Bring the chicken to room temperature.

Oil a grill or grill pan to and heat to medium-high heat. Place the chicken on the grill and cook until the chicken is firm to the touch and the juices run clear, 2 minutes on each side.

Serve garnished with the parsley and the drizzle.

COOK'S NOTE: Giving your chicken a good pounding will allow the flavor to infuse into the meat in as little as 15 minutes of marinating time.

PER SERVING: Calories: 222; Total Fat: 10 g (1 g saturated, 4 g mono-unsaturated); Carbohydrates: 4 g; Protein: 27 g; Fiber: 2.5 g; Sodium: 248 mg

STORAGE: Store in an airtight container in the refrigerator for up to 5 days.

ZA'ATAR

2 tablespoons dried thyme

2 tablespoons sesame seeds, toasted

1 tablespoon dried sumac

1 tablespoon dried oregano

1 tablespoon dried marjoram

CHICKEN

1 tablespoon extra-virgin olive oil

1 tablespoon za'atar

1/4 teaspoon lemon zest

1/4 teaspoon sea salt

1/4 teaspoon freshly ground black pepper

4 skinless, boneless organic chicken breasts or thighs

2 tablespoons finely chopped fresh parsley, for garnish

My Everything Drizzle (page 178)

Braised Chicken and Earthy Root Vegetables

MAKES 4 SERVINGS • PREP TIME: 20 minutes • COOK TIME: 35 minutes

This recipe reminds me of Thanksgiving, where root vegetables hold court to the delight of all. They are very grounding, and their time deep in the soil fills them with brain-healthy minerals and vitamins. Potassium, magnesium, iron, folate, and vitamins A and C all contribute to better brain functioning. Then there's the taste: a hale and hearty fullness, enhanced by thyme, sage, and rosemary. Swap out the chicken for turkey and call it Thanksgiving in a pot.

8 boneless, skinless organic chicken thighs

Sea salt

Freshly ground black pepper

3 tablespoons extra-virgin olive oil

1 yellow onion, diced small

1 medium fennel bulb, cut into $^1/_2$-inch dice

2 teaspoons minced garlic

Pinch of red pepper flakes

1 teaspoon dried thyme

$^1/_2$ teaspoon dried sage

$^1/_4$ teaspoon chopped fresh rosemary

1 medium sweet potato, peeled and cut into 1-inch chunks

1 large carrot, peeled and cut into 1-inch chunks

1 medium parsnip, peeled, and cut into 1-inch chunks

3 tablespoons dried cranberries

4 cups Old-Fashioned Chicken Stock (page 46) or store-bought organic stock

3 tablespoons freshly squeezed orange juice

2 teaspoons grated orange zest

Freshly squeezed lemon juice

3 tablespoons finely minced flat-leaf parsley, for garnish

Pat the chicken dry and season with salt and pepper. Heat 2 tablespoons of the olive oil in a Dutch oven or heavy-bottomed soup pot over medium-high heat. Add the chicken, working in batches if necessary, and cook until well browned on each side, about 3 minutes per side. Transfer to a plate.

Decrease the heat to medium and add the last tablespoon of olive oil. Add the onion, fennel, and a pinch of salt and sauté until soft and slightly golden, about 5 minutes. Add the garlic and red pepper flakes and sauté for 1 minute. Add thyme, sage, and rosemary and stir. Add the sweet potato, carrot, parsnip, cranberries, and $^1/_4$ teaspoon of salt and stir to combine. Pour in $^1/_4$ cup of the stock to deglaze the pot, stirring to loosen any brown bits. Stir in a pinch of salt and cook until the liquid is reduced by half. Add $1^3/_4$ more cups of stock, 2 tablespoons of the orange juice, and the orange zest. Decrease the heat to medium-low, cover, and simmer for 10 minutes.

Increase the heat to medium-high and add the remaining 2 cups of the stock. Snuggle the chicken down among the vegetables and simmer, uncovered, until the chicken is fully cooked, about 10 minutes. Stir in the remaining tablespoon of orange juice and lemon juice to taste.

Transfer to a serving dish, garnish with parsley, and serve.

COOK'S NOTE: Pan searing allows proteins to brown while leaving the interior nice and moist. The keys to achieving this are to not overcrowd the pan and to not turn the meat before it is ready to release from the pan. Put your largest pieces in first, as they'll take a bit longer to cook.

PER SERVING: Calories: 395; Total Fat: 21.5 g (5 g saturated, 12 g mono-unsaturated); Carbohydrates: 20 g; Protein: 34 g; Fiber: 8 g; Sodium: 350 mg

STORAGE: Store in an airtight container in the refrigerator for up to 3 days or freeze for up to 1 month.

Baked Chicken
WITH MINTED CHIMICHURRI

MAKES 4 SERVINGS · PREP TIME: 20 minutes plus up to 2 hours to marinate · COOK TIME: 40 minutes

Chicken isn't given its due as a brain food, and that's an omission worth correcting. It's absolutely loaded with tryptophan, which can boost mood and make sleep come easier. It's also high in vitamin B3 (aka niacin), which the Chicago Health and Aging Project, in a study of more than 3,700 individuals, found may slow cognitive decline. Here we take chicken thighs and jazz 'em up with a tantalizing mint chimichurri: with its South American roots, it's one of my go-to sauces for chicken.

Put the chicken in a large bowl with 6 tablespoons of the chimichurri and toss to coat. Cover with plastic wrap and marinate in the refrigerator for 45 minutes or up to 2 hours.

Preheat the oven to 400°F. Line a rimmed baking sheet with parchment paper.

Wipe off any of the marinating chimichurri. Place the chicken on the prepared baking sheet skin side up and season with the salt and pepper. Bake for 40 minutes or until the juices run clear and an instant-read thermometer inserted into the thickest part of a thigh reaches 160°F.

Transfer the chicken to a serving platter and drizzle a few tablespoons of the chimichurri over it. Serve, with the rest of the chimichurri on the side.

8 pasture-raised bone-in, skin-on chicken thighs

1 1/2 cups Minted Chimichurri (page 177)

1/2 teaspoon sea salt

1/4 teaspoon freshly ground black pepper

PER SERVING: Calories: 140; Total Fat: 7 g (2 g saturated, 0 g monounsaturated); Carbohydrates: 4.5 g; Protein: 14 g; Fiber: 0.5 g; Sodium: 426 mg

STORAGE: Store in an airtight container in the refrigerator for up to 5 days.

Mediterranean Roasted Chicken

MAKES 6 SERVINGS · PREP TIME: 15 minutes · COOK TIME: 1 hour 10 minutes (includes resting meat)

Roast chicken has so much potential, and here's how to reach it. First, there's your basic bird: mine are always organic or pasture-raised, which guarantees a quantum leap in flavor and nutrients such as vitamin A and omega-3 fatty acids. Then it all depends upon how you massage your bird. Rub deep and make sure you get the herbs and spices under the skin. Then finish with a dollop because your bird needs a little accessorizing to hit the "yum" mark.

1 (4$\frac{1}{2}$- to 5-pound) organic chicken

1 teaspoon ground paprika

$\frac{1}{2}$ teaspoon ground turmeric

$\frac{1}{4}$ teaspoon ground coriander

$\frac{1}{4}$ teaspoon ground cumin

$\frac{1}{4}$ teaspoon ground cinnamon

$\frac{1}{4}$ teaspoon red pepper flakes

1$\frac{1}{2}$ teaspoons sea salt

1 teaspoon grated fresh ginger, plus 3 inches unpeeled fresh ginger, halved lengthwise

3 cloves garlic, peeled

1 cinnamon stick

1 lemon, halved

2 teaspoons freshly squeezed lemon juice

My Everything Drizzle (page 178)

Preheat the oven to 400°F.

Pat the chicken dry with paper towels. Stir the paprika, turmeric, coriander, cumin, cinnamon, and red pepper flakes together. Divide the mixture in half and stir 1 teaspoon of the salt into one half. Rub the salted spice mixture all over the outside of the chicken. Sprinkle the remaining $\frac{1}{2}$ teaspoon of salt inside the chicken.

With your palm facing downward, use your first three fingers to gently lift the skin on both sides of the breast to loosen it from the meat. Rub the remaining spice mixture and the grated ginger under the skin of each side of the breast, massaging the seasonings lightly into the meat. Place the garlic cloves, cinnamon stick, and ginger pieces inside the cavity. Squeeze the lemon halves into the cavity, then insert the rinds.

Place the chicken on a roasting rack in a glass or ceramic baking dish, breast side up. Roast until a meat thermometer reads 160°F when inserted in the thigh and the juice from the meat runs clear, about 1 hour.

Let the chicken rest for at least 10 minutes before carving. Just before serving, pour 2 teaspoons of lemon juice all over the chicken and serve with My Everything Drizzle.

VARIATION: Here is a western Mediterranean spice blend: remove the cinnamon and ginger. In place of the turmeric, paprika, coriander, and cumin, use $\frac{1}{2}$ teaspoon of dried thyme, $\frac{1}{4}$ teaspoon of rosemary, $\frac{1}{2}$ teaspoon of fennel seeds, and $\frac{1}{4}$ teaspoon of sage. Serve with Olive and Sun-Dried Tomato Tapenade (page 184) or Parsley Pistou (page 175).

PER SERVING: Calories: 427; Total Fat: 31 g (9 g saturated, 13 g monounsaturated); Carbohydrates: 2 g; Protein: 33.5 g; Fiber: 0.5 g; Sodium: 433 mg

STORAGE: Store in a covered container in the refrigerator for 3 to 5 days.

Turkish Lamb Sliders

MAKES 4 SERVINGS • PREP TIME: 1 hour (includes resting meat) • COOK TIME: 6 minutes

Travel the world and you'll often find that lamb is the red meat of choice, and with good reason. Its high B12 profile makes it a great brain booster, while its leanness makes it low in cholesterol. Then there's lamb's malleable texture, which makes it the perfect starting point for building an awesome slider. My mixture here is positively Mediterranean, with pistachios, thyme, parsley, mint and a hit of anti-inflammatory spices. Put the Yogurt Tahini Raita (page 185) on top and you'll never, ever go near ketchup again. I promise. And since they're sliders (two ounces of lamb) versus a burger (big, bigger, biggest, *boom!*), it doesn't take more than one or two to get the protein hit you crave without feeling gorged.

Place the grated onion in a small strainer and press with the back of a spoon to drain any excess liquid. In the bowl of a food processor combine the onion, pistachios, garlic, cumin, cinnamon, salt, pepper, cayenne, thyme, parsley, and mint and process until finely ground.

Put the lamb in a large bowl, then add the onion and nut mixture. Mix it around with your hands until the ingredients are well distributed. Shape into 8 patties about 1/2 inch thick. Place the patties on a sheet pan and let rest in the fridge for 30 minutes to an hour.

Preheat the broiler and place the rack four of five inches below the heating element.

Place the sheet pan with the patties under the broiler and cook for about 3 minutes. Flip and cook the other side for another 3 minutes. Patties will still be pink in the middle.

Serve the sliders on lettuce leaves with a dollop of the Yogurt Tahini Raita.

COOK'S NOTE: These sliders can be made a day in advance. The minimum resting time of 30 to 60 minutes allows the proteins to relax after being worked.

PER SERVING: Calories: 223; Total Fat: 19 g (6 g saturated, 7 g mono-unsaturated); Carbohydrates: 2.5 g; Protein: 11 g; Fiber: 1 g; Sodium: 135 mg

STORAGE: Store cooked sliders in the refrigerator tightly wrapped in plastic wrap for up to 3 days, or uncooked in the freezer tightly wrapped for 1 month.

1/2 yellow onion, grated

1/2 cup pistachios

3 cloves garlic, coarsely chopped

1 teaspoon ground cumin

1/4 teaspoon ground cinnamon

1/2 teaspoon sea salt

1/4 teaspoon freshly ground black pepper

Pinch of cayenne

1 teaspoon minced fresh thyme

2 tablespoons coarsely chopped parsley

2 tablespoons coarsely chopped fresh mint

1 pound ground organic lamb

Butter or romaine lettuce leaves

1/2 cup Yogurt Tahini Riata (page 185)

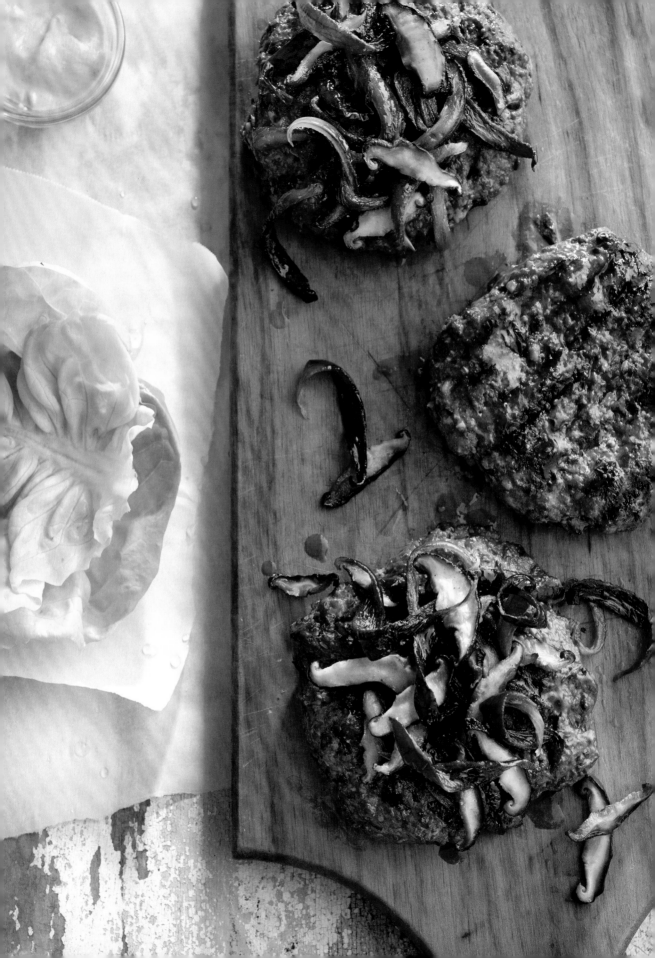

Grilled Bison Burgers
WITH CARAMELIZED ONIONS AND CRISPY SHIITAKES

MAKES 4 SERVINGS · PREP TIME: 15 minutes · COOK TIME: 30 minutes

I know it says bison here, but that lean meat (bison=buffalo) is really just a great excuse to hold a mushroom-a-palooza while getting a load of brain-boosting B12. First we mix the bison with chopped-up cremini mushrooms. Then on top go a few crispy shiitakes that have been tossed with smoked paprika and olive oil. In between? Caramelized onions (*ummmmmm...*). Put it all on a lily pad of butter lettuce and it tastes like a Tower of Umami! The mushrooms also provide a hit of hard-to-find vitamin D, which University of Kentucky researchers found plays an important role in reducing oxidative damage in the brain that impacts learning.

Preheat oven to 375°F. Line a baking sheet with parchment.

Place the shiitakes in a bowl and drizzle with 2 tablespoons of the olive oil, salt, and paprika, tossing until evenly coated. Arrange the mushrooms in a single layer on the prepared sheet pan and roast until crisp and browned, about 20 minutes.

To caramelize the onions, heat the remaining 2 tablespoons of olive oil in a large skillet over medium-high heat. When the oil starts to shimmer, add the onion and a generous pinch of salt. Cook slowly, stirring occasionally, until the onion is caramelized and very soft, 20 to 25 minutes. Remove from the pan.

To make the burgers, place the bison, cremini mushrooms, parsley, and black pepper in a large bowl. Rinse the anchovies and, in a small bowl or mortar and pestle, mash them to a paste with 1/2 teaspoon of salt. Using the same skillet as the onions, heat the 1 teaspoon of oil over medium heat. Add the garlic and red pepper flakes to the mashed anchovies, stirring to combine. Sauté for 1 minute then transfer this mixture to the large bowl with the meat and mushroom mixture. Using your hands, gently mix until everything is well combined. Shape into 4 equal-size patties.

Heat a grill or grill pan to medium-high heat and lightly coat with a neutral-flavored oil. Grill the patties, turning once, for 3 minutes per side.

Serve each patty on a lettuce leaf topped with some caramelized onion and crispy shiitake mushrooms.

8 ounces shiitake mushrooms, stems removed and thinly sliced

4 tablespoons extra-virgin olive oil

1/4 teaspoon sea salt

1/4 teaspoon smoked paprika

1/2 large red onion, sliced

BURGERS

1 pound ground bison

3 ounces cremini mushrooms, stemmed and finely processed in a food processor

3 tablespoons coarsely chopped parsley

1/2 teaspoon freshly ground black pepper

2 skinless, boneless anchovies

Sea salt

1 teaspoon extra-virgin olive oil

1 1/2 tablespoons minced garlic

Pinch of red pepper flakes

4 butter lettuce leaves, washed and dried

CONTINUED

Grilled Bison Burgers, *continued*

COOK'S NOTES: When you mix the bison with the other ingredients, use a light hand. If you overwork the meat, the burgers will be tough.

When it comes to caramelizing onions, patience is a virtue. During cooking, the onions slowly change appearance, turning from translucent to a deep golden brown as they release their yummy sugars. Keep in mind that onions will cook down to less than one-third their original volume as they caramelize. You'll want to stir the onions, but resist the urge. The key is to cook them slow and low. After about 20 minutes, the onions should begin to wilt and take on a golden hue, and if you have the patience to let them go ten minutes longer, they'll take on a deeper color and become even sweeter. Caramelized onions hold well in the fridge and add a lot of flavor to other dishes, so make extra.

PER SERVING: Calories: 368; Total Fat: 25 g (6 g saturated, 15 g mono-unsaturated); Carbohydrates: 12 g; Protein: 26 g; Fiber: 3 g; Sodium: 264 mg

STORAGE: Store the patties tightly wrapped in plastic wrap in the refrigerator for up to 3 days or, uncooked, tightly wrapped in the freezer for 1 month.

Rosemary and Thyme–Smothered Lamb Chops

MAKES 4 SERVINGS · PREP TIME: 10 minutes plus 30 minutes to marinate · COOK TIME: 6 minutes

Lamb chops were always a special occasion in our house. So much so that mom would dress them up in little paper chef's hats that went over the ends of the bones (I think, in her heart, she was an origami lover). I love lamb chops, not only for the taste, but also the size; they epitomize my belief that you only need a little bit of meat to satisfy a craving while (in the case of lamb) getting a full shot of brain-boosting B12 and protein. The key is going with grass-fed lamb (it's less gamey) and using a dollop (here, I suggest you use My Everything Drizzle, page 178). And there's no Wizard-of-Oz-emerald-green mint jelly here; instead, the lamb is rubbed with a generous amount of garlic, rosemary, and thyme.

In a small bowl, combine the garlic, rosemary, thyme, mustard, olive oil, and zest. Season each lamb chop with the salt and pepper. Gently massage each lamb chop with the rub and let them sit at room temperature for at least 30 minutes.

Grill the chops at medium-high heat or broil for about 3 minutes a side for medium rare (see Cook's Note), until an instant-read thermometer registers an internal temperature of 140°F. Allow to rest for 5 minutes, then serve with a dollop of My Everything Drizzle.

COOK'S NOTE: To broil, place the chops on a generously oiled broiler pan or wire rack set atop a large, rimmed baking sheet and place 4 to 5 inches from the heating element.

PER SERVING: Calories: 300; Total Fat: 15 g (4.5 g saturated, 9 g mono-unsaturated); Carbohydrates: 1.5 g; Protein: 35 g; Fiber: 0 g; Sodium: 172 mg

STORAGE: Store in an airtight container in the refrigerator for up to 3 days.

8 cloves of garlic, minced to a paste

2 teaspoons minced rosemary

1 tablespoon minced fresh thyme

2 teaspoons Dijon mustard

2 teaspoons extra-virgin olive oil

1 teaspoon lemon zest

8 lamb chops, well trimmed

Sea salt

Freshly ground black pepper

My Everything Drizzle (page 178)

Thai It Up Steak Salad

MAKES 6 SERVINGS · PREP TIME: 15 minutes · COOK TIME: 20 minutes

The lesson here is that a little beef goes a long way. What people crave is the taste and texture of beef, not to be overwhelmed by it, and this dish satisfies that need by turning beef into a supporting player. The headliners here are the veggies and the dressing: think a big band combo filled with horns (that's the lime and chili paste dressing), a rollicking rhythm section (shredded cabbage, peppery watercress, crunchy cucumber), and silkily dressed pitch-perfect backup singers (the cellophane noodles). Add meat and bring down the house!

DRESSING

1/3 cup freshly squeezed lime juice

2 teaspoons lime zest

1 tablespoon Grade B maple syrup

1 tablespoon freshly grated ginger

1 1/2 tablespoons Thai fish sauce

1 1/2 to 2 teaspoons chili paste

1/4 cup mild olive oil or grapeseed oil

1 1/2 pounds flank steak, trimmed

1 tablespoon olive oil

1/2 teaspoon sea salt

1/4 teaspoon freshly ground pepper

3 1/2 ounces cellophane (bean thread) or rice stick noodles

2 cups arugula or mixed greens

1 cup thinly sliced red cabbage

1 cup loosely packed basil leaves

1 cup loosely packed cilantro leaves

1 cup loosely packed mint leaves

1 red bell pepper, stemmed, seeded, and thinly sliced

1 English cucumber, peeled, seeded and thinly sliced

1/4 cup cashews (optional)

In a small bowl, whisk together the lime juice, zest, maple syrup, ginger, fish sauce, and chili paste. Slowly whisk in the oil until well combined.

Put the steak in a shallow dish; rub with 1 tablespoon olive oil, season with salt and pepper, and rub with about half the dressing; reserve the remaining dressing. Let it marinate for 10 to 15 minutes. Heat a grill or grill pan to high heat. Generously oil the grate or grill pan and grill the steak until an instant-read thermometer registers 135°F for medium-rare, about 3 to 4 minutes per side depending on the thickness.

Transfer the steak to a cutting board and cover loosely with foil; allow it to rest for 5 minutes. Slice the steak diagonally across the grain into thin pieces and drizzle with 2 tablespoons of the reserved dressing.

Meanwhile, prepare the noodles according to the package directions. When the noodles are cooked, rinse them with cold water, and drain them well. Transfer them to a large bowl and toss with 1 tablespoon of the dressing.

Add the arugula, cabbage, basil, cilantro, mint, bell pepper, cucumber, and noodles and toss with the remaining dressing (you should have about 2 tablespoons left). Divide the salad evenly onto 6 plates and arrange the steak over the salad. Sprinkle each serving with cashews.

COOK'S NOTE: Keep your eye on the grill. Grass-fed beef is leaner than grain-fed beef and will dry out if overcooked. For perfect taste and texture, cook to rare or medium-rare. If you like your beef well done, then cook it at a very low temperature.

PER SERVING: Calories: 376; Total Fat: 19 g (4 g saturated, 11 g monounsaturated); Carbohydrates: 25 g; Protein: 27 g; Fiber: 2.5 g; Sodium: 443 mg

STORAGE: Store in an airtight container in the refrigerator for up to 3 days.

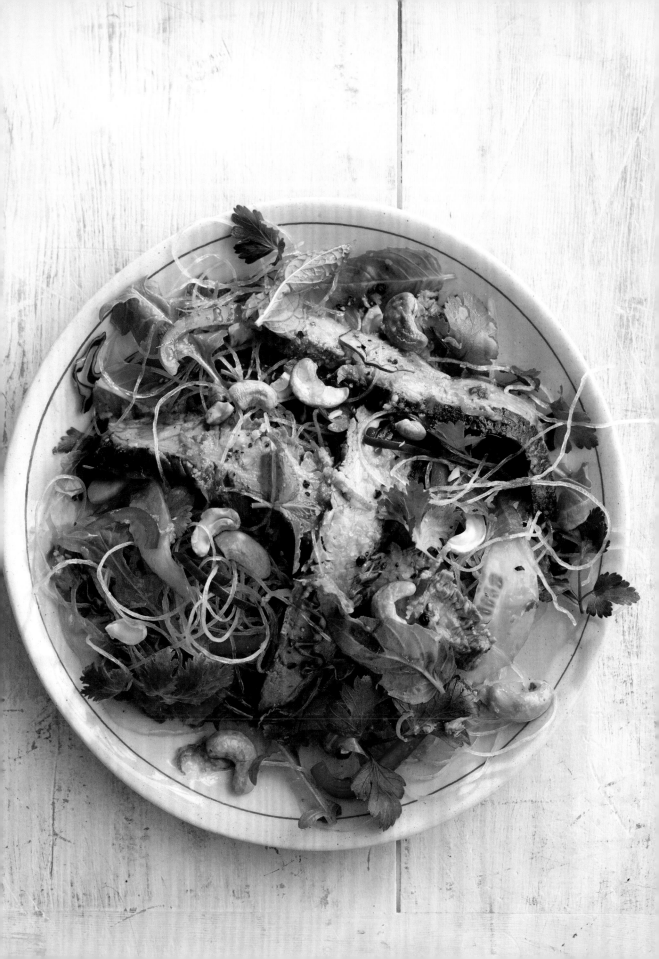

Almost Better Than Nana's Brisket

MAKES 6 SERVINGS · PREP TIME: 20 minutes · COOK TIME: 3 hours

I've called this "almost" better out of respect to my nana, but just between us . . . let's say it's even Stephen. Nana really understood that a tender brisket required braising patience or you'd end up with the table version of beef jerky. The whole braising process invites experimentation. There's something about a stew pot that screams "C'mon! Show me what else you've got!!" My mother used to throw beer in the pot, but Nana had a secret ingredient that made her brisket stand out from ordinary fare—ginger and a touch of molasses. My version involves deglazing the pot with red wine and eventually adding lots of immune-boosting aromatics, including garlic, cinnamon, caraway seeds, fennel seeds, and ginger, which is a great digestive aid. The meat comes out as tender as a grandmother's goodnight kiss on the head. Nana, this one's for you. Thanks for showing me the way. This brisket goes great with Ginger Lime Sweet Potato Mash (page 100), Rutabaga and Potato Mash-Up (page 95), or Celery Root Mash-Up (page 94).

2 pounds organic lean grass-fed brisket

Sea salt

Freshly ground black pepper

1 1/2 tablespoons extra-virgin olive oil

1 large yellow onion, coarsely chopped

3 carrots, peeled and diced

3 stalks celery, diced

2 cloves garlic, chopped

1/4 teaspoon caraway seeds

1/4 teaspoon ground cinnamon

2 teaspoons freshly grated ginger, or 1/2 teaspoon ground ginger

1/4 teaspoon crushed fennel seeds

Pinch of red pepper flakes

1 tablespoon tomato paste

1 cup red wine

1 cup crushed canned tomatoes

4 to 6 cups Nourishing Bone Broth (page 67) or store-bought organic stock

1/2 teaspoon unsulfured or blackstrap molasses

Preheat the oven to 300°F.

Allow the brisket to come to room temperature, trim excess fat, and thoroughly dry with a paper towel. This ensures that your meat browns more evenly and doesn't steam. Season the beef all over with salt and pepper.

Heat the olive oil in a Dutch oven or other braising pot over medium heat. When the oil starts to shimmer, add the brisket. Cook for 6 minutes without moving the meat until it's browned and easily lifts from the bottom of the pan. Turn the meat over and brown the second side for 6 minutes more. Remove the beef and transfer it to a large plate.

In the same pot over medium heat, add the onion, carrots, celery, and 1/4 teaspoon of salt. Sauté until golden, about 6 minutes. Add the garlic, caraway, cinnamon, ginger, fennel, and pepper flakes and continue sautéing for 1 minute more. Stir in the tomato paste, then add the wine, stir the pot to scrape up any browned bits, and continue to cook until the wine has almost evaporated.

Return the brisket to the pot and add the tomatoes and enough broth to just cover the brisket. Cover the pot and bring to a slow boil, then remove the brisket from the stove top and place it in the oven. Cook for 2 hours and 15 minutes. Remove the brisket from the oven and transfer to a cutting board. Remove 2 cups of liquid to a small saucepan, bring to a boil, and reduce the sauce by half. Then stir in the molasses.

Meanwhile, slice the brisket thinly against the grain, aligning your knife so it's perpendicular to the fibers of the meat. Transfer the sliced meat back to the original pot and simmer on the stove top for an additional 30 minutes. It's ready when a fork comes out easily without resistance. Serve with generous spoonfuls of sauce.

COOK'S NOTE: Sometimes you need a thermometer to know when meat is ready, but here all you need is a fork. This brisket cooks slow and long, and it's not ready until your fork slides through the meat without any resistance. If it's still fighting back, sit down and read another chapter of that great book you've been meaning to get back to; check again in 15 minutes.

PER SERVING: Calories: 328; Total Fat: 10 g (3 g saturated, 5.5 g mono-unsaturated); Carbohydrates: 17 g; Protein: 35 g; Fiber: 4 g; Sodium: 417 mg

STORAGE: Store in an airtight container for 5 days or freeze up to 1 month.

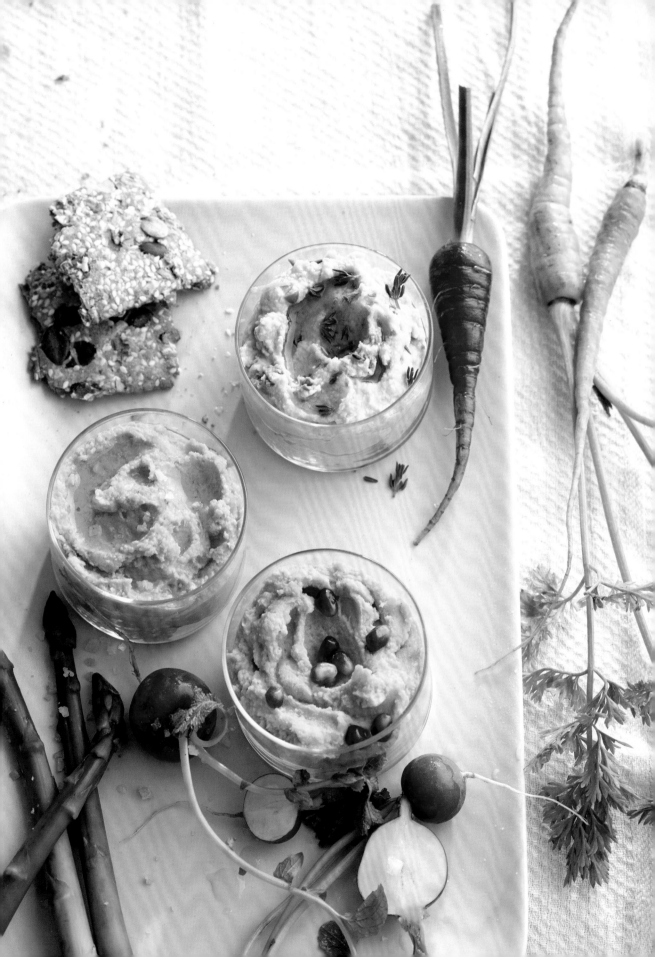

CHAPTER 7

Anytime Foods

As the name implies, anytime foods are designed to be enjoyed . . . whenever. They let you eat small amounts throughout the day, a pattern that is ideal for blood sugar regulation. You'll also eat the right kinds of foods—those that promote a slow absorption of sugar into the bloodstream. To do otherwise is to promote high levels of insulin in the body, which can lead to insulin resistance and the inability of the brain to properly metabolize sugar. Insulin resistance is linked to a load of brain issues, including depression and cognitive decline. So when those pre- or post-lunchtime hunger cravings get your stomach growling and your mind whirling, you have a choice: head for the vending machine (Warning, Will Robinson! Warning!) or reach into your bag for something far tastier and healthier. In this chapter, you'll find lots of nutrients packed into little packages (Apple Pie–Spiced Walnuts and Raisins, page 161; Coconut Curry Cashews, page 160), complete proteins (Dolled-Up Quinoa, page 142), fast fish (#SuperiorMoodSardines, page 138), and quick pick-me-up snacks (Toasty Spiced Pumpkin Seeds, page 159; five different sweet and savory muffins, pages 150 to 155). There are twenty-two recipes in all, and with good reason. I want to provide you with a huge rotation of delicious anytime foods that are portable, perfect for work, play, or even a stay-at-home day.

Wild Salmon Scramble

MAKES 4 SERVINGS • PREP TIME: 10 minutes • COOK TIME: ABOUT 5 minutes

I love the idea of scrambles because you can get a ton of goodies into one dish. This scramble is perfect if you've got some serious mental gymnastics coming up during the day (like taking a final). Here we're taking two ounces of wild smoked sockeye salmon, a few pasture-raised eggs, and goat cheese—all great protein foods, with the salmon kicking in omega-3s—adding some dill and scallion, scrambling it all up and serving it over ripe tomatoes. You could take a picture, it's so pretty. But you better have a fast shutter speed, cause these scrambles get eaten up in a flash.

2 ripe red tomatoes, sliced

Sea salt

Freshly ground black pepper

4 pasture-raised eggs

1 tablespoon minced fresh dill, or 1 teaspoon dried

1 tablespoon extra-virgin olive oil

1 1/2 ounces goat cheese

2 ounces smoked wild sockeye salmon, broken into 1/2-inch pieces

1 tablespoon minced scallion, both green and white parts

1 tablespoon minced fresh chives, for garnish

Set out 4 plates and put two slices of tomato in the center of each plate. Sprinkle each serving with a small pinch of salt and a grind of pepper.

In a bowl, combine the eggs, salt, pepper and dried dill, if using, then whisk until frothy. Heat the olive oil in an 8- to 10-inch skillet over medium-high heat, until hot. Add the eggs and decrease the heat to low. Using a spatula, fold the eggs, pulling them off the side of the skillet toward the center, about a minute. When halfway set, add in the goat cheese and stir it in. When nearly set, but still wet, turn off the heat and fold in the salmon, fresh dill if using, and some of the scallion.

Evenly divide the eggs and salmon and mound them on top of the tomatoes slices. Garnish with the chives and the remaining scallions and serve immediately.

COOK'S NOTE: I like to cook my eggs low and slow. Low heat and slow cooking keeps them from becoming rubbery.

PER SERVING: Calories: 159; Total Fat: 11 g (4 g saturated, 5 g mono-unsaturated); Carbohydrates: 5 g; Protein: 9 g; Fiber: 1 g; Sodium: 223 mg

STORAGE: Not applicable

Sweet Potato Hash

MAKES 4 SERVINGS • PREP TIME: 20 minutes • COOK TIME: 30 minutes

It's funny how time changes a food's reputation. In the nineteenth century, there were diners called hash houses, and the cooks therein were known as hashslingers. Move forward a hundred years or so, and hash isn't slumming any more. Connoisseurs of a fine hash are glad to invest the chopping time involved because the results are downright yummy. Roasted sweet potatoes combine with sautéed onions, garlic, a fistful of herbs, and Italian or turkey sausage for a simply heavenly hash.

Preheat oven to 425°F. Line 2 rimmed baking pans with parchment paper.

Put the sweet potatoes in a large bowl. Add 2 tablespoons of the olive oil, $1/2$ teaspoon of salt, and $1/4$ teaspoon of pepper and toss until evenly coated. Spread the sweet potatoes evenly in a single layer and roast for 25 minutes or until tender. Remove from the oven and set aside.

While the sweet potatoes are roasting, heat a large, heavy skillet over medium heat and add the remaining 2 tablespoons of olive oil. When the oil is shimmering, add the onion and a pinch of salt and sauté until translucent , about 4 minutes. Stir in the garlic, rosemary, sage, fennel seed, and red pepper flakes and sauté until aromatic, about 30 seconds. Add the sausage, break it apart, and cook until it's no longer pink, about 5 minutes. Add the sweet potatoes and spinach, stirring until well combined, and the spinach is just wilted.

Divide the hash onto four plates. Give a grind of black pepper and a pinch of salt to each.

1 sweet potato, peeled and cut into $1/4$-inch dice

$1/4$ cup extra-virgin olive oil

Sea salt

Freshly ground black pepper

$1/2$ onion, diced

3 cloves garlic, minced

$1^1/2$ teaspoons minced fresh rosemary, or $1/4$ teaspoon dried

$1^1/2$ teaspoons minced fresh sage, or $1/4$ tablespoon dried

$1/4$ teaspoon crushed fennel seed

Pinch of red pepper flakes

8 ounces sweet Italian turkey or chicken sausage, casing removed

3 cups baby spinach

PER SERVING: Calories: 488; Total Fat: 26 g (5 g saturated, 13 g mono-unsaturated); Carbohydrates: 41.5 g; Protein: 26 g; Fiber: 6 g; Sodium: 822 mg

STORAGE: Store leftover hash in an airtight container in the refrigerator for up to 4 days.

Sunshine Up Baked Eggs

MAKES 4 SERVINGS · PREP TIME: 10 minutes · COOK TIME: 25 minutes

There's something about sunny-side up eggs that make me smile. It's just that happy old yellow yolk, sitting neatly in its own white canvas, that gets me going. The only thing I don't like about sunny-side ups is when they come off the griddle, full of grease. But we avoid that here by baking the eggs in little ramekins filled with a sautéed mix of chard, onion, and garlic. On top go some chopped parsley, olives, and tomatoes, and when all is said and done you've got yourself a little cup of sunshine.

1 bunch chard, washed and dried

1 tablespoon extra-virgin olive oil

4 scallions, minced

Sea salt

1 teaspoon minced garlic

Pinch of red pepper flakes

Pinch of freshly grated nutmeg

1/4 cup crumbled organic feta cheese (optional)

4 organic eggs

8 cherry tomatoes, quartered

8 kalamata olives, coarsely chopped

2 tablespoons basil chiffonade or 1 teaspoon minced fresh thyme, for garnish

2 tablespoons finely chopped parsley, for garnish

Preheat the oven to 350°F.

Remove the chard leaves and roughly tear them into bite-size pieces. Chop the remaining stems into 1/2-inch pieces. Heat the olive oil in a sauté pan over medium heat, then add the scallions, chard stems, and a pinch of salt and sauté until the scallions are translucent, about 4 minutes. Stir in the garlic, red pepper flakes, and a pinch of salt and sauté for an additional 30 seconds, then stir in the chard and another pinch of salt and cook until tender, about another minute or two. Remove from the heat and stir in the nutmeg.

Lightly grease four 1-cup ramekins with olive oil. For each ramekin, spoon in one-fourth of the chard mixture, then sprinkle on one-fourth of the cheese. Gently crack 1 egg on top of the cheese, then sprinkle the tomatoes, olives, and a pinch of salt evenly over all 4 ramekins. Put the ramekins on a baking sheet and bake for 20 to 25 minutes, until the whites are set and opaque but the yolk is still runny.

Let cool for 3 minutes, then run a knife or an offset spatula around the inside edge of each ramekin to loosen the eggs. Using your knife or spatula to help support the eggs, carefully transfer to a plate and sprinkle with the basil and parsley and serve immediately.

COOK'S NOTES: To avoid a watery end product, make sure the greens are dried well prior to adding them to the sauté pan.

When you transfer the greens to the ramekin, don't pack them down too tightly. You want to allow space for the egg to filter down into the container. This allows the eggs and greens to hold together better when you transfer them to the plate.

PER SERVING: Calories: 120; total Fat: 9.5 g (2.6 g saturated, 5.0 g monounsaturated); Carbohydrates: 6 g; protein: 7 g; Fiber: 2 g; sodium: 285 mg

STORAGE: Not applicable

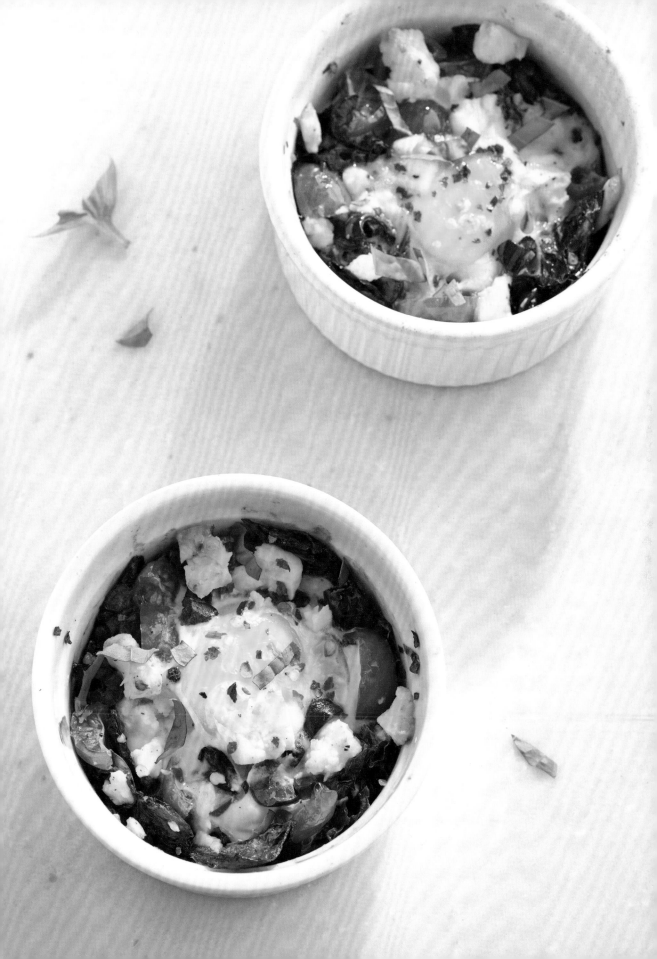

#SuperiorMoodSardines

This is my ode to the tiny fish of my youth. We had a young family friend from Norway who had Dusty Springfield hair and a taste for sardines. She'd dress them up just so and the two of us would go to town on open-faced sardine tea sandwiches. I've never lost my taste for this omega-3 powerhouse, and whenever I want to improve my mood, I reach for a can of sardines the way other people gravitate toward a tin of tuna. Here, I work in a little lemon juice and lemon zest to brighten up the taste, along with diced celery and pickle, parsley, thyme, and olive oil. The only thing I don't do is mush the whole thing up so it looks like cat food. Just a little flaking of the sardines with a fork is enough to make this both look and taste ridiculously appealing, so much so that I think they should inspire their own Twitter hashtag.

Freshly squeezed lemon juice

1 teaspoon lemon zest

1 teaspoon Dijon mustard

1 teaspoon extra-virgin olive oil

1/8 teaspoon sea salt

Grind of black pepper

2 small scallions, minced

1 tablespoon finely diced cornichon, or 1 teaspoon pickle relish

1 tablespoon finely diced celery

1 tablespoon coarsely chopped fresh parsley

2 teaspoons minced fresh thyme

1 (3³/4-ounce) can sardines, drained

6 leaves of endive, romaine or butter lettuce, washed and dried

Mix 4 teaspoons of lemon juice, the zest, mustard, olive oil salt, pepper, scallions, cornichon, celery, parsley, and thyme together in a bowl. Add the sardines and flake them into chunky pieces with a fork. Stir gently to combine. Taste; you may want to add a pinch of salt or a generous squeeze of lemon juice. Scoop into the endive leaves and serve.

PER SERVING: Calories: 135; Total Fat: 9 g (2 g saturated, 4.5 g mono-unsaturated); Carbohydrates: 2 g; Protein: 12.5 g; Fiber: 0.5 g; Sodium: 5.93 mg

STORAGE: Store in an airtight container in the refrigerator for up to 2 days.

Falafel Mini Sliders

MAKES 4 SERVINGS • PREP TIME: 20 minutes • COOK TIME: 30 minutes

Lovers of falafel have a conundrum. The taste is outstanding, but traditional falafel is deep-fried. It all comes down to the kind of fats you want in your diet, and here we avoid all the grease by going with a baked version instead. Just twenty minutes and you've got a load of adorable, healthy bites: falafel is the perfect host for a load of brain-boosting herbs and spices including turmeric, a potent anti-inflammatory. The yogurt-tahini sauce is a fantastic topping. Now you can have your falafel stress-free. I love these served with Lemon Tahini Dressing (page 181) and Kale Quinoa Salad with Red Grapes (page 89).

Preheat the oven to 375°F. Line a rimmed baking sheet with parchment paper.

Put the chickpeas in a bowl and stir in a spritz of lemon juice. Set aside. In the bowl of a food processor, combine the bell peppers, scallions, parsley, zest, tahini, 2 tablespoons plus 1 teaspoon of lemon juice, the olive oil, garlic, ginger, salt, turmeric, paprika, cumin, coriander, and cinnamon. Pulse about 15 times, until combined. Add the chickpeas and pulse another 25 times, until you see it start to form a ball.

Put about 2 tablespoons of the mixture in your palm and shape it into a little patty; place on the prepared baking sheet. Bake the patties for about 25 minutes or until they begin to get dry and crisp on the outside. They will firm up more as they cool.

COOK'S NOTES: If you want to cook just a few patties, pop them in your toaster oven.

To freeze these falafel sliders cooked or uncooked, stack them with parchment paper between the patties. Wrap the entire stack first in plastic wrap, then in foil. The parchment paper makes it easy to remove the desired number of sliders from the bundle. Once thawed, cooked patties can be reheated at 350°F for 15 minutes and uncooked patties can be baked as above, at 375°F for 22 to 25 minutes. They don't need to be turned.

PER SERVING: Calories: 159; Total Fat: 7 g (1 g saturated, 2 g mono-unsaturated); Carbohydrates: 18 g; Protein: 7.5 g; Fiber: 4 g; Sodium: 124 mg

STORAGE: Store well wrapped in the refrigerator for up to 5 days. To freeze, see the Cook's Notes.

2 cups cooked chickpeas, or 1 (15-ounce) can, rinsed

Freshly squeezed lemon juice

1/4 cup coarsely diced red bell pepper

1/4 cup sliced scallions

1/2 cup coarsely chopped fresh parsley

1 1/2 teaspoons lemon zest

3 tablespoons tahini

1 tablespoon extra-virgin olive oil

2 cloves garlic, coarsely chopped

1 teaspoon coarsely chopped fresh ginger

1/2 teaspoon sea salt

1/4 teaspoon ground turmeric

1/2 teaspoon paprika

1/4 teaspoon ground cumin

1/4 teaspoon ground coriander

1/8 teaspoon ground cinnamon

1 lemon, cut into wedges, for garnish

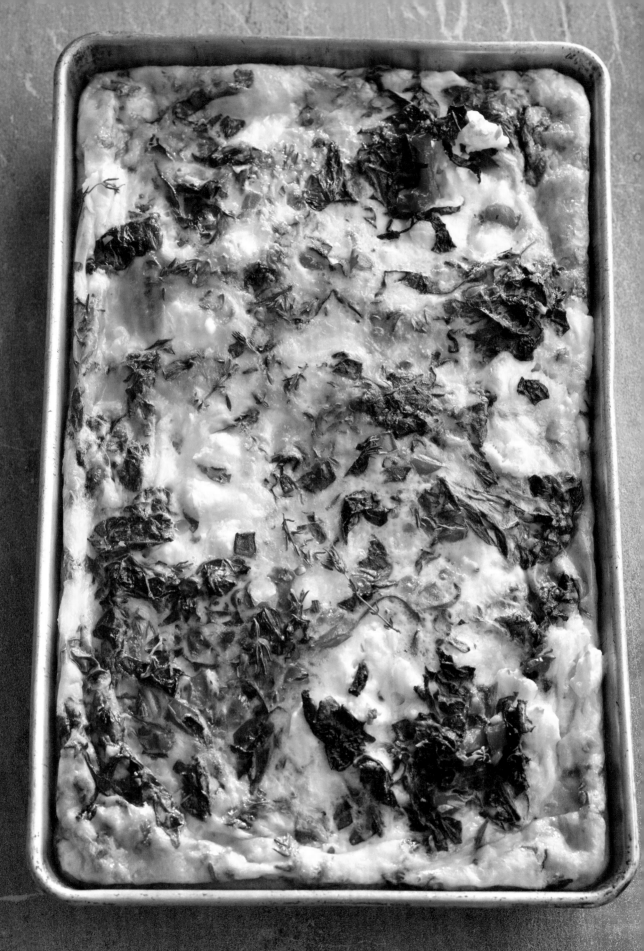

Triple Greens Frittata

MAKES 6 SERVINGS · PREP TIME: 15 minutes · COOK TIME: 40 minutes

A frittata is an Italian omelet but, unlike the French version, you don't have to figure out how to do that funky half-flip with the eggs in the pan. Frittatas bake, and in Italy they're often eaten at room temperature: they really are a good on-the-go food. The eggs are also a great binder for the greens, which include kale, chard, and spinach. Add some red bell pepper, marjoram, thyme, and feta, and you've got a super protein hit for lunch on the go—just the thing to keep your brain working optimally throughout the day.

Preheat the oven to 375°F. Lightly oil a 6 by 8-inch baking dish.

Heat the oil in a large skillet over medium heat. When it's shimmering, add the bell pepper and a pinch of salt and sauté for 3 minutes. Add the garlic and red pepper flakes and sauté until fragrant, another 30 seconds or so. Stir in the kale and another pinch of salt and continue to sauté for 5 minutes. Add the chard and spinach, and one more pinch of salt, sautéing until the greens are wilted and tender, about 5 minutes more. Remove from the heat and add a few gratings of nutmeg, stirring to combine.

Whisk the eggs, scallions, marjoram, thyme, 1/2 teaspoon of salt, and the pepper together in a large bowl. Lay the cooked greens along the bottom of the prepared dish and top them with the crumbled feta. Pour the egg mixture over and bake until the eggs are just set, 25 to 30 minutes.

PER SERVING: Calories: 169; Total Fat: 12 g (3.5 g saturated, 6.5 g monounsaturated); Carbohydrates: 6.5 g; Protein: 8g; Fiber: 1 g; Sodium: 388 mg

STORAGE: Store, tightly wrapped, in the refrigerator for up to 2 days.

2 tablespoons extra-virgin olive oil

1/2 cup diced red bell pepper

Sea salt

2 cloves garlic, minced

Pinch of red pepper flakes

1 cup tightly packed, finely chopped kale

2 cups tightly packed, finely chopped chard

2 cups tightly packed, finely chopped spinach

Freshly grated nutmeg

10 organic eggs

2 scallions, minced

2 tablespoons chopped fresh marjoram

1 tablespoon chopped fresh thyme

1/4 teaspoon freshly ground black pepper

2 ounces crumbled feta

Dolled-Up Quinoa

MAKES 4 SERVINGS · PREP TIME: 6 minutes · COOK TIME: 20 minutes

Quinoa sometimes gets a bad rap, but that's more often than not a case of user error. It has to be given a quick bath before going into the pot, otherwise its natural resins have a bitter taste. Now that you know better, there's no excuse for not diving into this amazing teeny grain, which resembles couscous. Quinoa is a complete protein, meaning it contains all the essential amino acids the brain needs. It also has the right mix of fiber, making for a slow burn as opposed to a simple carb blast. Did I mention it also makes a perfect backdrop for a light dish? Here quinoa complements saffron, shallots, ginger, and slivered almonds.

1 teaspoon warm water

1/4 teaspoon saffron

2 tablespoons extra-virgin olive oil

2 tablespoons finely diced shallot

2 teaspoons grated fresh ginger

Sea salt

1 cup quinoa, rinsed

1 1/2 cups Classic Magic Mineral Broth Classic (page 44), store-bought organic stock, or water

1 tablespoon freshly squeezed orange juice

1 tablespoon freshly squeezed lemon juice

1 teaspoon lemon zest

2 tablespoons finely chopped fresh parsley

2 tablespoons sliced almonds, toasted, for garnish

Combine the warm water and saffron in a small bowl and set aside.

Heat the olive oil in a saucepan over medium heat, then add the shallot, ginger, and a pinch of salt and sauté for about 1 minute. Then add the quinoa and stir to combine. Add the saffron and its water and give a quick stir. Stir in the broth and 1/2 teaspoon of salt and bring to a boil. Lower the heat to medium–low, cover, and simmer for about 18 to 20 minutes, stirring once halfway through the cooking, until the liquid has been absorbed and the quinoa is tender.

Remove from the heat and let it sit, covered for 10 minutes. Fluff the quinoa with a fork, then add the orange and lemon juices, zest, and parsley and fluff again. Taste; you may want to add a couple of pinches of salt and another spritz or two of lemon juice. Sprinkle with the toasted almonds and serve.

COOK'S NOTE: If you do not have saffron, then substitute 1/4 teaspoon of turmeric for a beautiful color.

PER SERVING: Calories: 277; Total Fat: 12 g (1 g saturated, 6 g mono-unsaturated); Carbohydrates: 34 g; Protein: 8 g; Fiber: 12 g; Sodium: 284 mg

STORAGE: Store in the refrigerator in an airtight container for 3 days.

Ginger Scented Forbidden Rice

MAKES 4 SERVINGS • PREP TIME: 5 minutes (after soaking rice overnight) • COOK TIME: 30 minutes

What once was forbidden is now fabulous and available to all. This rice, with it's deep royal purple color, nutty flavor, and alleged longevity properties, was the exclusive property of Chinese emperors: during the Ming Dynasty it was referred to as "tribute rice." I can't say whether it really will help you live longer, but the rice's anthocyanins (the source of its rich color) are a super antioxidant, which protects brain health. The twist in this recipe is infusing the rice with a subtle, relaxing ginger scent.

2 ($1/2$-inch) slices rinsed unpeeled fresh ginger, plus 1 teaspoon minced fresh ginger

$1/2$ teaspoon sea salt

1 cup forbidden rice, soaked in water overnight

In a 2-quart pot over high heat, bring 2 cups of water, sliced ginger, minced ginger, and salt to a boil, then stir in the rice. Cover, lower the heat, and simmer for 30 minutes, until the water is all absorbed and the rice is tender.

Remove the ginger slices and serve.

PER SERVING: Calories: 174; Total Fat: 2 g (0.5 g saturated, 0.6 g monounsaturated); Carbohydrates: 38 g; Protein: 5 g; Fiber: 3.5 g; Sodium: 306 mg

STORAGE: Store in an airtight container in the refrigerator for up to 2 days.

Bejeweled Forbidden Rice Salad

MAKES 6 SERVINGS • PREP TIME: 5 minutes (after soaking rice overnight) • COOK TIME: 30 minutes

This is certainly a case for visuals drawing you to the plate. Served with salmon, this rice—an indigo delight—pops like a painting, beckoning you to come closer, closer . . . and that first bite seals the deal. The rice and bell pepper play delightfully against the creaminess of the avocado, while the mint and cilantro roll all around your mouth like pinballs, blasting taste here, there, and everywhere. This salad enchants all the senses—and the rice is a whole grain as well, feeding the mind in more ways than one.

2 cups water

1/2 teaspoon sea salt

1 cup forbidden rice

1/4 cup Cilantro Lime Vinaigrette (page 166)

1/2 cup diced celery

1/4 cup diced red bell pepper

1 scallion, minced

1/4 cup finely chopped fresh mint

1 avocado, cut in 1/2-inch dice

In a 2-quart pot over high heat, combine 2 cups of water and the salt and bring to a boil, then stir in the rice. Cover, lower the heat to medium low, and simmer for 20 to 25 minutes, then check the rice. It should be tender, but still with a nice chew. Fluff the rice with a fork, then transfer it to a bowl and allow it to cool.

Add the vinaigrette and toss to combine. Then mix in the celery, bell pepper, scallion, and mint. Top with avocado just before serving.

PER SERVING: Calories: 235; Total Fat: 13 g (2 g saturated, 9 g mono-unsaturated); Carbohydrates: 29 g; Protein: 4 g; Fiber: 5 g; Sodium: 181 mg

STORAGE: Store in an airtight container without avocado in the refrigerator for up to 2 days. Re-dress the salad before serving; you will have 1/4 cup of dressing left over from making the vinaigrette in the first place.

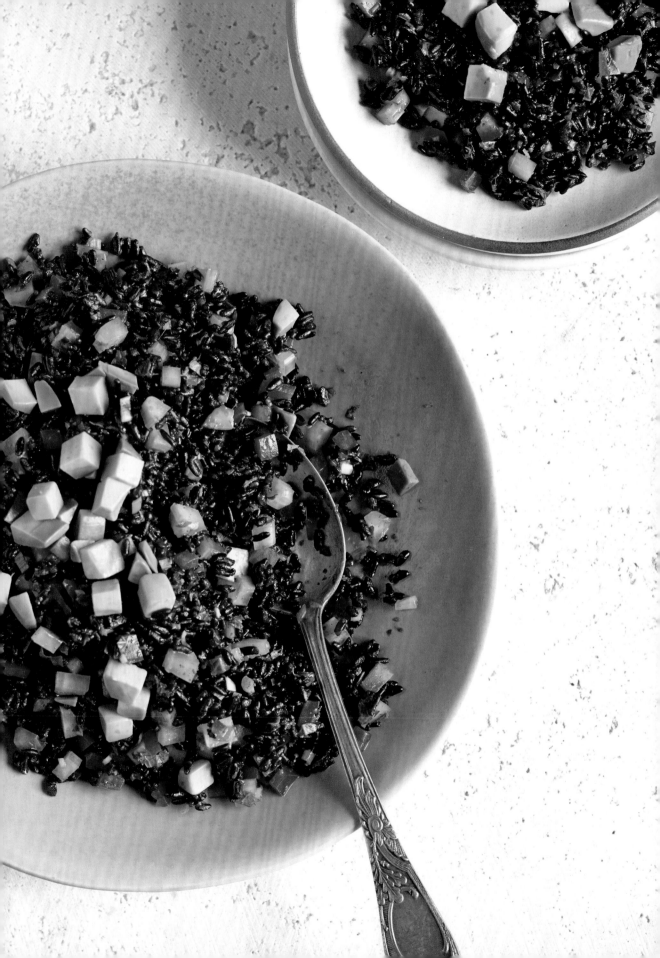

Double Red Pepper Hummus

MAKES 3 CUPS • PREP TIME: 5 minutes • COOK TIME: Not applicable

Roasted red bell pepper gives this hummus a bit of a twist. In and of themselves, red bell peppers are a little mellow on the heat for my taste, so I've cranked up the flame a tad by adding a pinch of cayenne. Cayenne wakes up both your taste buds and your brain; a major compound in cayenne, capsaicin, has been shown to elevate endorphins and mood. Who knows? A few nibbles and you might be ready take a belly dancing class.

2 cup cooked chickpeas, or 2 (15-ounce cans), rinsed

Freshly squeezed lemon juice

Sea salt

$1/2$ cup coarsely chopped roasted red peppers

Extra-virgin olive oil

1 tablespoon tahini

1 clove garlic, coarsely chopped

2 tablespoons water

$1/4$ teaspoon cayenne pepper

1 tablespoon fresh basil chiffonade (optional)

In a bowl, mix the chickpeas with a spritz of lemon juice and a pinch of salt. Combine the chickpeas, roasted red peppers, 2 tablespoons of lemon juice, 2 tablespoons of olive oil, tahini, garlic, $1/2$ teaspoon of salt, 2 tablespoons of water, and cayenne pepper in a food processor and process until smooth. Taste; You may want to add a pinch more salt and/or squirt of lemon. Transfer to a small bowl and garnish with basil and a drizzle of olive oil.

COOK'S NOTE: There's a nice kick of cayenne when this is served right away. However, the cayenne mellows after it's been refrigerated, so you may want to add a spritz of lemon and another pinch of cayenne just to wake this hummus up.

To freeze hummus, fill an airtight container, leaving a $1/2$ an inch to allow for expansion during freezing. To retain the moisture of the dip during freezing, pour 2 teaspoons of olive oil over the hummus to form a protective seal. Transfer the hummus from the freezer to the refrigerator one day before you are ready to use it, as it takes several hours to thaw. Stir the hummus well before serving. Taste; you may need to add a squeeze of lemon or a pinch salt to wake it up from its deep sleep in the freezer.

PER SERVING: Serving Size: $1/4$ cup; Calories: 152; Total Fat: 8 g (1 g saturated, 4 g monounsaturated); Carbohydrates: 16.5 g; Protein: 6 g; Fiber: 4.5 g; Sodium: 139 mg

STORAGE: Store in an airtight container in the refrigerator for up to 7 days or in the freezer for up to 4 months.

Meyer Lemon and Caper Hummus

MAKES 3 CUPS · PREP TIME: 5 minutes · COOK TIME: Not applicable

It's nice to have understanding neighbors. I've often joked that I moved to Northern California for the Meyer lemons, but when I first got here I didn't have a Meyer lemon tree. Fortunately, my neighbors did, so every once in a while they'd look out their rear window and see some strange little pixie filling her apron with their lemons. Eventually, I got a teeny tree, which somehow turned into four, and now I have more lemons than I know what to do with. Hence, Meyer lemon caper hummus. This hummus is bright and a delight, because the lemons are actually sweet, as if they were crossed with an orange. Actually, I kind of miss sneaking into my neighbors' yard, even if it was pilfering with permission. There's something about a liberated lemon that adds to the excitement of the dish.

In a bowl, mix the chickpeas with a spritz of lemon juice and a pinch of salt. Combine the chickpeas, $1/4$ cup of lemon juice, lemon zest, capers, 2 tablespoons of olive oil, tahini, garlic, water, and $1/2$ teaspoon of salt in the bowl of a food processor and process until smooth, about a minute. Taste; you may want to add a pinch more salt or squirt of lemon. Transfer to a small bowl and garnish with thyme and a drizzle of olive oil.

PER SERVING: Serving Size: $1/4$ cup; Calories: 180; Total Fat: 8 g (4 g saturated, 1 g monounsaturated); Carbohydrates: 16 g; Protein: 7 g; Fiber: 7 g; Sodium: 630 mg

STORAGE: Serve in an airtight container in the refrigerator for up to 7 days or in the freezer for up to 4 months. For instructions on how to thaw the hummus, see Cook's Notes, page 146.

2 cups cooked chickpeas, or 2 (15-ounce) cans, rinsed

Freshly squeezed Meyer lemon juice

Sea salt

2 teaspoons lemon zest

2 tablespoons capers, rinsed

Extra-virgin olive oil

1 tablespoon tahini

1 teaspoon coarsely chopped garlic

3 tablespoons water

1 teaspoon minced thyme (optional), for garnish

Curry Spiced Sweet Potato Hummus

MAKES ABOUT 2 CUPS • PREP TIME: 5 minutes • COOK TIME: 12 minutes

Hummus has been popular since at least the thirteenth century, where it appeared in an Egyptian cookbook. And as far as its being too exotic to make, well, that's really not the case. Hummus is simply a mix of pureed chickpeas, lemon juice, and tahini, which is just ground-up sesame seeds (fortunately for your brain, they're full of zinc). Hummus is a great foundation for experimentation, and here I've pumped up the colors and flavors by introducing sweet potatoes topped with pomegranate seeds and mint. There's an earthy, mellow taste to this creamy hummus that resonates on a deep level, with cumin, curry, and ginger spicing providing just the right level of *ahhhhhh* . . . .

8 ounces sweet potatoes, peeled and cut into $^1/_2$-inch cubes

Sea salt

1 cup cooked chickpeas, or 1 (15-ounce) can, rinsed

Freshly squeezed lemon juice

Extra-virgin olive oil

1 tablespoon tahini

1 teaspoon curry powder

1 teaspoon ground cumin

1 teaspoon ground ginger

3 tablespoons water

3 tablespoons pomegranate seeds (see Cook's Notes), for garnish

1 tablespoon minced mint, for garnish

Set a steamer basket in a pot, then fill with enough water to hit just below the bottom of the basket. Add the sweet potatoes with a sprinkle of salt. Bring to a boil over high heat and steam, covered, for 10 to 12 minutes or until tender.

In a bowl, mix the chickpeas with a spritz of lemon juice and a pinch of salt. Combine the sweet potatoes, chickpeas, $2^1/_2$ tablespoons of lemon juice, 2 tablespoons of olive oil, tahini, curry powder, cumin, ginger, $^1/_2$ teaspoon of salt, and water in the bowl of a food processor and process until smooth. Taste; you may want to add a pinch more salt or squirt of lemon. Transfer to a small bowl and garnish with pomegranate seeds, mint, and a drizzle of olive oil.

COOK'S NOTES: Here's a quick trick for removing pomegranate seeds from the fruit. Cut the pomegranate in half crosswise. Then, working over a large bowl, hold one half with the cut side facing down into the bowl. Give the uncut side of the fruit a few good whacks with the back of a large wooden spoon to release the seeds, letting them fall into the bowl. If no pomegranate seeds are available, then a drizzle of pomegranate molasses will do.

Served immediately, this hummus is smooth and dippable. After refrigerating, the potatoes soak up moisture and it becomes more of a spread. For instructions on how to freeze and thaw, see Cook's Notes, page 146.

PER SERVING: Serving Size: $^1/_4$ cup; Calories: 229; Total Fat: 12 g (2 g saturated, 7 g monounsaturated); Carbohydrates: 26 g; Protein: 6 g; Fiber: 6 g; Sodium: 237 mg

STORAGE: Store in an airtight container in the refrigerator for up to 5 days or in the freezer for up to 1 month.

Tart Cherry and Chocolate Crunch

MAKES ABOUT 10 CUPS · PREP TIME: 10 minutes · COOK TIME: 30 minutes

This is so good, it might leave you speechless. I mean, what's not to love? Almonds, pecans, walnuts, dark chocolate chips, dark cherry, coconut . . . are you dizzy yet? I'm not trying to brag, but when we gave a friend of ours some of this granola, he took one bite and asked, "Will it travel?" When we said "Yes," he said, "Good . . . I'm taking it to Honduras with me!" I hope the customs folks there don't ask for a nibble. We put some into a jar on the top shelf of my kitchen to see how long it would hold up; turns out it held up longer than we did. We got to a week before we devoured it all. And believe me, that was *after* employing a lot of willpower.

Preheat over to 325°F. Line a rimmed baking sheet with parchment paper.

In a large bowl, whisk together the maple syrup, orange zest, coconut oil, salt, and vanilla. Pulse the almonds, pecans, and walnuts together in the bowl of a food processor until the pieces are the size of raisins. Add the nuts, oats, chocolate chips, coconut, and cherries to the bowl and mix until everything is well coated.

Spoon the mixture onto the baking sheet and, with wet hands or a small piece of parchment paper, spread and press it into an even layer about $1/4$ inch thick, filling the baking sheet. Tuck in any loose pieces on the edges.

Bake for about 30 minutes or until golden brown. Start checking at 20 minutes and turn the sheet if necessary. Allow to cool completely before breaking into pieces.

COOK NOTE: If you are sensitive to gluten, use gluten-free oats.

PER SERVING: Serving Size: $1^{1}/2$ cups; Calories: 275; Total Fat: 18 g (7 g saturated, 5 g monounsaturated); Carbohydrates: 26 g; Protein: 5 g; Fiber: 4 g; Sodium: 22 mg

STORAGE: Store in an airtight container for up to a month.

$1/2$ cup Grade B maple syrup

1 teaspoon orange zest

$1/4$ cup coconut oil, melted

$1/4$ teaspoon sea salt

1 teaspoon vanilla

1 cup coarsely chopped almonds

1 cup coarsely chopped pecans

1 cup coarsely chopped walnuts

2 cups old-fashioned rolled oats

$3/4$ cup bittersweet chocolate chips

$2/3$ cup unsweetened shredded coconut

1 cup dried tart cherries

Olive, Lemon Zest, and Thyme Muffins

MAKES 24 MINI MUFFINS • PREP TIME: 15 minutes • COOK TIME: 15 minutes

Muffins—in this case mini muffins—are an outstanding delivery system for a load of different tastes. I liked that idea, but wanted to get beyond the lard-filled, wheat-laden muffins so common to the American palate. My answer was to focus on almond flour, aka almond meal. It's easy to work with, gluten-free, and high in relaxing magnesium, and it increases production of dopamine, a neurotransmitter involved in stabilizing mood. It makes its appearance here and in the next four recipes: each of these muffins, some savory, some sweet, are nutrient-dense, meaning a few mini bites are all you need to fill you up, anytime, anywhere.

At first you might not think olives and almonds would go together, but I've always noticed that, when I put out a dish of olives and a bowl of almonds as snacks, people tend to go back and forth between both. So, I just glued them together in this muffin, along with some lemon zest and thyme. Trust me on this one; it works.

2 cups almond meal

$1/2$ teaspoon sea salt

$1/4$ teaspoon freshly ground black pepper

$1/2$ teaspoon baking soda

3 large organic eggs

$3^1/2$ tablespoons extra-virgin olive oil

$1^1/2$ teaspoons lemon zest

$1/2$ tablespoon freshly squeezed lemon juice

$1/2$ tablespoon water

$1^1/2$ teaspoons Grade B maple syrup

12 kalamata olives, chopped

1 tablespoon minced fresh thyme

6 tablespoons finely chopped parsley

Preheat the oven to 350°F. Oil a mini muffin tin or line it with muffin papers.

In a bowl, mix together the almond meal, salt, pepper, and baking soda. In another bowl, whisk together the eggs, olive oil, lemon zest, lemon juice, water, and maple syrup. Add the wet ingredients to the dry ones and stir well to combine. Then stir in the kalamata olives, thyme, and parsley. Fill each muffin cup with about 2 tablespoons of batter.

Bake for 13 to 15 minutes, until a toothpick comes out clean.

COOK'S NOTES: Mini muffin tins come in a variety of sizes. I prefer using tins whose cups have a wide base, around $1^1/2$ inches in diameter. Don't despair if you can't find that exact size, as most anything will work.

To prevent the muffins from sticking to the bottom of the pan, make sure you grease the cups really, really, well. Then, after baking you must exercise patience and allow the muffins to cool completely before removing them from the tin.

PER SERVING: Serving Size: 2 mini muffins. Calories: 173; Total Fat: 15.5 g (2 g saturated, 4 g monounsaturated); Carbohydrates: 5 g; Protein: 6 g; Fiber: 2 g; Sodium: 204 mg

STORAGE: Store in an airtight container for up to 5 days

Cranberry, Orange, and Apricot Muffins

MAKES 24 MINI MUFFINS • PREP TIME: 15 minutes • COOK TIME: 15 minutes

Whenever you use dried fruits, the tastes are intensified. Here the surprise fruit is apricot, whose slight sweetness plays perfectly off of cranberry's tartness. This muffin has a lot of crunchy-chewy going on, which many people enjoy.

Preheat the oven to 350°F. Oil a mini muffin tin or line with muffin papers.

In a bowl, mix together the almond meal, salt, and baking soda. In another bowl, whisk together the eggs, olive oil, maple syrup, lemon juice, water, and vanilla. Add the wet ingredients to the dry and stir well to combine. Then stir in the cranberries, apricots, and orange zest. Fill each muffin cup with about 2 tablespoons of batter.

Bake for 13 to 15 minutes, until a toothpick comes out clean.

PER SERVING: Serving Size: 2 mini muffins. Calories: 161; Total Fat: 13 g (1 g saturated, 2 g monounsaturated); Carbohydrates: 8 g; Protein: 6 g; Fiber: 2 g; Sodium: 114 mg

STORAGE: Store in an airtight container for up to 5 days.

2 cups almond meal

1/4 teaspoon sea salt

1/2 teaspoon baking soda

3 large organic eggs

2 tablespoons olive oil

2 tablespoons Grade B maple syrup

1/2 tablespoon freshly squeezed lemon juice

1/2 tablespoon water

1 teaspoon vanilla extract

3 tablespoons coarsely chopped fresh, frozen, or dried cranberries

3 tablespoons minced dried apricot

1 1/2 teaspoons orange zest

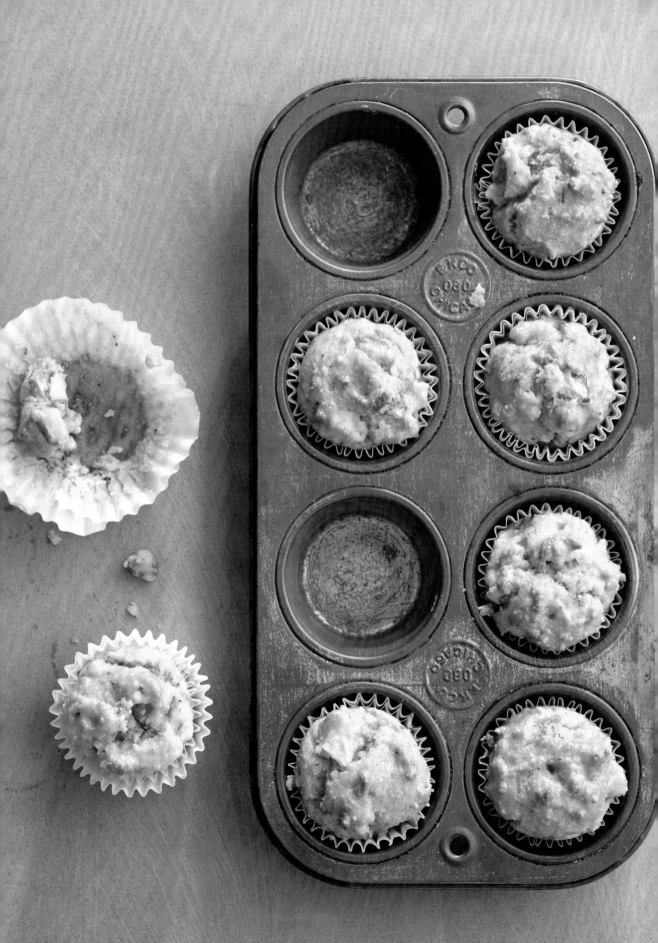

Rosemary and Pear Muffins

MAKES 24 MINI MUFFINS · PREP TIME: 15 minutes · COOK TIME: 15 minutes

Here's a surprising combination. Rosemary tends to be assertive, while pears go mellow; together they make an unbeatable team. This muffin is as Mediterranean as they come. Draw a direct line from Florence to Provence, and this puppy's flavor lands right in the middle.

Preheat the oven to 350°F. Oil a mini muffin tin or line it with muffin papers.

In a bowl, mix together the almond meal, salt, pepper, and baking soda. In another bowl, whisk together the eggs, olive oil, lemon juice, water, and maple syrup. Add the wet ingredients to the dry and stir well to combine. Then add in the pears, walnuts, and rosemary. Fill each muffin cup with about 2 tablespoons of batter.

Bake for 13 to 15 minutes, until a toothpick comes out clean.

PER SERVING: Serving Size: 2 mini muffins. Calories: 182; Total Fat: 16 g (2 g saturated, 4 g monounsaturated); Carbohydrates: 7 g; Protein: 6 g; Fiber: 2 g; Sodium: 147 mg

STORAGE: Store in an airtight container for up to 5 days.

2 cups almond meal

$1/2$ teaspoon sea salt

$1/4$ teaspoon freshly ground black pepper

$1/2$ teaspoon baking soda

3 large organic eggs

$3^1/_2$ tablespoons extra-virgin olive oil

$1/2$ tablespoon lemon juice

$1/2$ tablespoon water

$1^1/_2$ teaspoon Grade B maple syrup

$1/2$ cup diced ripe Anjou pear

3 tablespoons chopped walnuts

$1^1/_2$ teaspoons finely minced fresh rosemary

Apple, Cinnamon, Ginger, and Currant Muffins

MAKES 24 MINI MUFFINS · PREP TIME: 15 minutes · COOK TIME: 15 minutes

This muffin reminds me of one of my mom's apple coffee cakes. Just add a cup of tea, and this is an absolute delight. The cinnamon acts as a warming spice, and is very comforting.

2 tablespoons plus 2 teaspoons olive oil

1/2 cup finely diced apple

1 teaspoon ground cinnamon

1/2 teaspoon ground ginger

2 cups almond meal

1/4 teaspoon sea salt

1/2 teaspoon baking soda

3 large organic eggs

2 tablespoons Grade B maple syrup

1/2 tablespoon freshly squeezed lemon juice

1/2 tablespoon water

1 teaspoon vanilla extract

2 tablespoons currants

Preheat the oven to 350°F. Oil a mini muffin tin or line with muffin papers.

In a small skillet over medium-high heat, add 2 teaspoons of the olive oil, then the apples and cook for 3 to 5 minutes, stirring occasionally, until the apples are soft. Remove the skillet from the heat, add the cinnamon and ginger, and stir until well combined and fragrant. Allow to cool while making batter.

In a bowl, mix together the almond meal, salt, and baking soda. In another bowl, whisk together the eggs, the remaining 2 tablespoons olive oil, maple syrup, lemon juice, water, and vanilla. Add the wet ingredients to the dry and stir well to combine. Stir in the apple mixture and the currants. Fill each muffin cup with about 2 tablespoons of batter. Bake for 13 to 15 minutes, until a toothpick comes out clean.

PER SERVING: Serving Size: 2 mini muffins. Calories: 162; Total Fat: 13 g (1 g saturated, 2 g monounsaturated); Carbohydrates: 9 g; Protein: 6 g; Fiber: 2 g; Sodium: 114 mg

STORAGE: Store in an airtight container for up to 5 days.

Raspberry, Lemon Zest, and Vanilla Muffins

MAKES 24 MINI MUFFINS • PREP TIME: 15 minutes • COOK TIME: 15 minutes

Vanilla and raspberry are definitely BFFs, as any ice cream lover can attest. Here they get a new friend, lemon zest, and darned if they don't all get along just swimmingly. If you don't have raspberries, blueberries or strawberries are also right at home in this muffin.

Preheat the oven to 350°F. Oil a mini muffin tin or line with muffin papers.

In a bowl, mix together the almond meal, salt, and baking soda. In another bowl, whisk together the eggs, olive oil, lemon juice, water, maple syrup, and vanilla. Add the wet ingredients to the dry and stir well to combine. Then stir in the raspberries, almonds, and lemon zest. Fill each muffin cup with about 2 tablespoons of batter. Bake for 13 to 15 minutes, until a toothpick comes out clean.

COOK'S NOTE: If you are using frozen raspberries, there is no need to thaw them. Simply give the berries a coarse chop and stir them into the batter.

PER SERVING: Serving Size: 2 mini muffins; Calories: 160; Total Fat: 13 g (1 g saturated, 2 g monounsaturated); Carbohydrates: 8 g; Protein: 6 g; Fiber: 3 g; Sodium: 114 mg

STORAGE: Store in an airtight container for up to 5 days.

2 cups almond meal

1/4 teaspoon sea salt

1/2 teaspoon baking soda

3 large organic eggs

2 tablespoons olive oil

1/2 tablespoon freshly squeezed lemon juice

1/2 tablespoon water

2 tablespoons Grade B maple syrup

1 1/2 teaspoons vanilla extract

1 cup fresh or frozen raspberries

3 tablespoons chopped toasted almonds

2 teaspoons lemon zest

Triple Triple Brittle

MAKES ABOUT 2 CUPS · PREP TIME: 5 minutes · COOK TIME: 30 minutes

This one reminded me of how Edison must've felt inventing the lightbulb: it took a lot of tries, but once I hit on the right formula, *shazam!* I knew we had a winner when I walked into my husband's office, brittle in hand. He was so deep in thought at his computer screen that he didn't even see me. I just said, "Gregg . . . open mouth." In went the brittle, his eyes still glued to the screen. "Gregg . . . close mouth. Chew." I was halfway down the hall when I finally heard his voice echo off the walls: "This is REALLY good!" And so it is, for the tongue and for the brain. The sesame seeds are full of zinc, the pumpkin seeds are like little mini antidepressants, and the sunflower seeds are loaded with vitamin E, which helps memory, learning, and overall mood.

1 cup raw pumpkin seeds

$3/4$ cup raw sunflower seeds

$1/4$ cup white or black sesame seeds

2 teaspoons ground cinnamon

1 teaspoon ground ginger

$1/2$ teaspoon ground allspice

$1/2$ teaspoon sea salt

$1/3$ cup Grade B maple syrup

1 teaspoon vanilla extract

Preheat the oven to 300°F. Line a rimmed baking sheet with parchment paper.

In a large bowl, combine the pumpkin seeds, sunflower seeds, sesame seeds, cinnamon, ginger, allspice, and salt, then add the maple syrup and vanilla and mix until well coated.

Spoon the mixture onto the prepared baking sheet and, with a spatula or a piece of parchment paper, pat and press the brittle into an even layer about $1/8$ inch thick. Press out the middle so it's slightly thinner than the edges, which will help prevent the outside edges from burning.

Bake for about 30 minutes or until golden brown. Remove from the oven and allow to cool completely. As it cools it will become crispy. Once the brittle has crisped up, break it into pieces.

COOK'S NOTES: If you have a small rolling pin—or a wine bottle for that matter—place a piece of parchment paper on top of the brittle mixture and use the rolling pin to create a nice even surface.

Warning! Sneaking a taste right out of the oven may burn your tongue.

If the brittle doesn't become crispy after it has cooled, put it back in the oven and bake for 8 to 10 minutes more.

PER SERVING: Serving Size: $1/2$ cup; Calories: 140; Total Fat: 10 g (1.5 g saturated, 0 g monounsaturated); Carbohydrates: 7.5 g; Protein: 4.5 g; Fiber: 1.25 g; Sodium: 90 mg

STORAGE: To keep the brittle crispy, store in a glass container on your counter for up to 2 weeks. It can be frozen in a ziplock bag for up to 3 months.

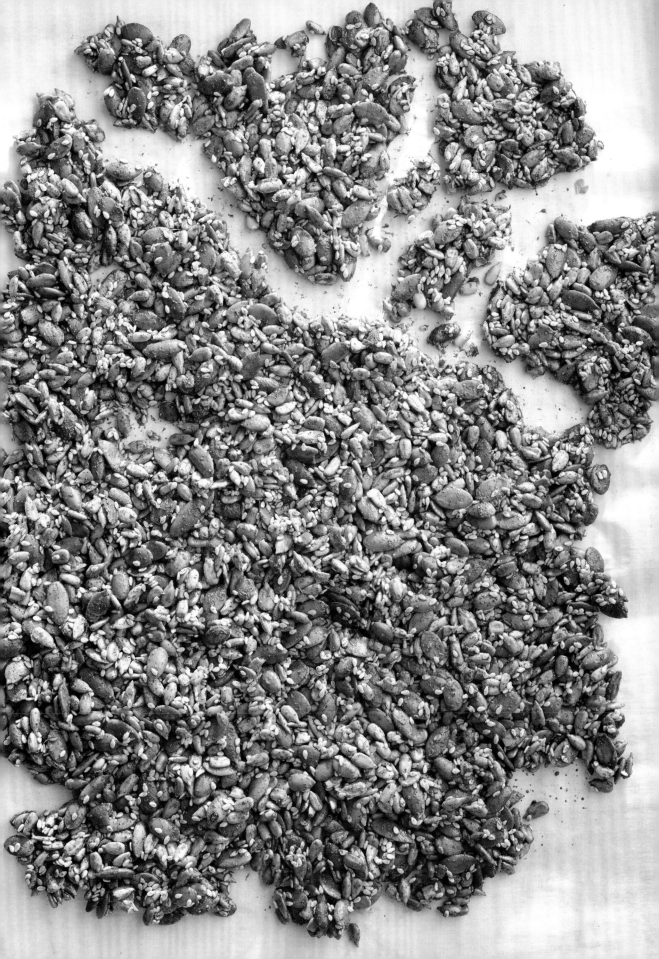

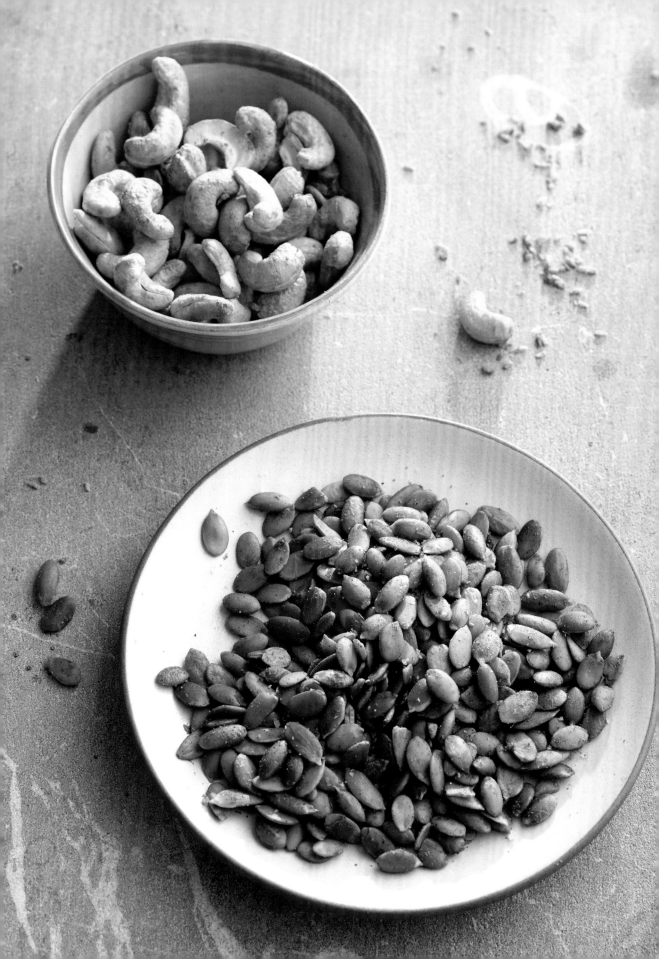

Toasty Spiced Pumpkin Seeds

MAKE ABOUT 1 CUP · PREP TIME: 5 minutes · COOK TIME: 8 minutes

I call pumpkin seeds nature's smallest antidepressant (next to a snowflake), and science backs me up; they contain glutamate, which produces GABA, a chemical that fights stress in the brain. They're also one of nature's finest portable snacks, and with this recipe there's no excuse for you not to have some in your purse or by your work desk. The seeds have a fantastic crunch and, tossed with cumin and coriander—two anti-inflammatory spices—a spectacular taste.

Preheat the oven to 350°F. Line a rimmed baking sheet with parchment paper.

Put all the ingredients in a bowl and stir until well combined. Spread evenly on the prepared baking sheet and bake for 7 to 8 minutes, until you can start to smell the spices. Check after 5 minutes to prevent burning. Allow to cool on the baking sheet.

COOK'S NOTE: Sometimes you need to use your ears in the kitchen. Once you hear the seeds start to pop, they're done.

1 cup raw pumpkin seeds

1 teaspoon extra-virgin olive oil

$1/4$ teaspoon sea salt

$1/2$ teaspoon ground cumin

$1/2$ teaspoon ground coriander

PER SERVING: Serving Size: $1/4$ cup; Calories: 132; Total Fat: 11.25 g (1.5 g saturated, 0.5 g monounsaturated); Carbohydrates: 2.75 g; Protein: 5.5 g; Fiber: 1.5 g; Sodium: 203 mg

STORAGE: Store in an airtight container for up to a month.

Coconut Curry Cashews

MAKES ABOUT 1 CUP · PREP TIME: 5 minutes · COOK TIME: 8 to 10 minutes

Nuts are little superstars when it comes to improving brain function; cashews are phenomenal at promoting good blood circulation so plenty of oxygen gets to the brain. That's the nutritional reason to eat cashews, but the taste alone should convince you. Here, I've deconstructed a complex curry to create a nice, quick, easy-to-make study snack, using shredded coconut, curry, a smidge of maple syrup, and, of course, the cashews. Take them to work and I promise your colleagues will be envious. So be a do-gooder and share.

1 teaspoon extra-virgin olive oil

1 teaspoon Grade B maple syrup

$1/2$ teaspoon curry powder

$1/2$ teaspoon ground ginger

$1/4$ teaspoon sea salt

1 cup cashews

2 teaspoons shredded coconut

Preheat the oven to 350°F. Line a rimmed baking sheet with parchment paper.

Put the olive oil, maple syrup, curry powder, ginger, and salt in a bowl and stir to combine. Add in the cashews and coconut and stir well with a spatula to evenly coat the cashews with the spices. Spread them evenly on the baking sheet. Roast in the oven for about 8 to 10 minutes.

COOK'S NOTE: When in doubt, take them out! Nuts will continue to cook after they have been removed from the oven.

PER SERVING Serving Size: $1/4$ cup; Calories: 229; Total Fat: 18 g (3.5 g saturated, 10 g monounsaturated); Carbohydrates: 13 g; Protein: 7 g; Fiber: 1.5 g; Sodium: 105 mg

STORAGE: Store in a container for up to 1 month. Freeze in an airtight container or ziplock bag for up to 3 months.

Apple Pie—Spiced Walnuts and Raisins

MAKES ABOUT 1 CUP • PREP TIME: 5 minutes • COOK TIME: 8 minutes

This is pure aromatherapy. There's nothing like the smell of baking apple pie to raise the spirits, so in this recipe I pulled together the spices that make apple pie special and gave them a new home—walnuts. Walnuts, with all their nooks and crannies, catch all the spices, especially after they're coated with a little olive oil and maple syrup (just writing this is making me practically salivate). Walnuts happen to be loaded with the omega-3 known as alpha-linolenic acid, which in animal studies exerted an antidepressant effect. Tossing them with plump raisins is the kicker.

Preheat the oven to 350°F. Line a rimmed baking sheet with parchment paper.

Put the olive oil, maple syrup, cinnamon, allspice, salt, and nutmeg in a bowl and stir to combine. Add in the walnuts and stir with a spatula to evenly coat the walnuts with the spices. Spread evenly on the prepared baking sheet. Roast in the oven for about 8 minutes, until you can begin to smell them. If adding raisins, toss them with the warm walnuts.

COOK'S NOTE: As soon as you start to smell that heavenly aroma wafting from the stove, it's time to remove the nuts from the oven. They will continue to cook as they cool.

The raisins will plump up as they are tossed with the warm nuts. Take a handful and eat these with sliced apples for a deconstructed, unbaked apple pie.

PER SERVING: Serving Size: $1/4$ cup; Calories: 227; Total Fat: 20 g (2 g saturated, 3.5 g monounsaturated); Carbohydrates: 11 g; Protein: 5 g; Fiber: 2.5 g; Sodium: 102 mg

STORAGE: Store in an airtight container for up to 1 month.

1 teaspoon extra-virgin olive oil

1 teaspoon Grade B maple syrup

$1/2$ teaspoon ground cinnamon

$1/4$ teaspoon ground allspice

$1/4$ teaspoon sea salt

$1/8$ teaspoon ground nutmeg

1 cup walnuts

3 tablespoons raisins (optional)

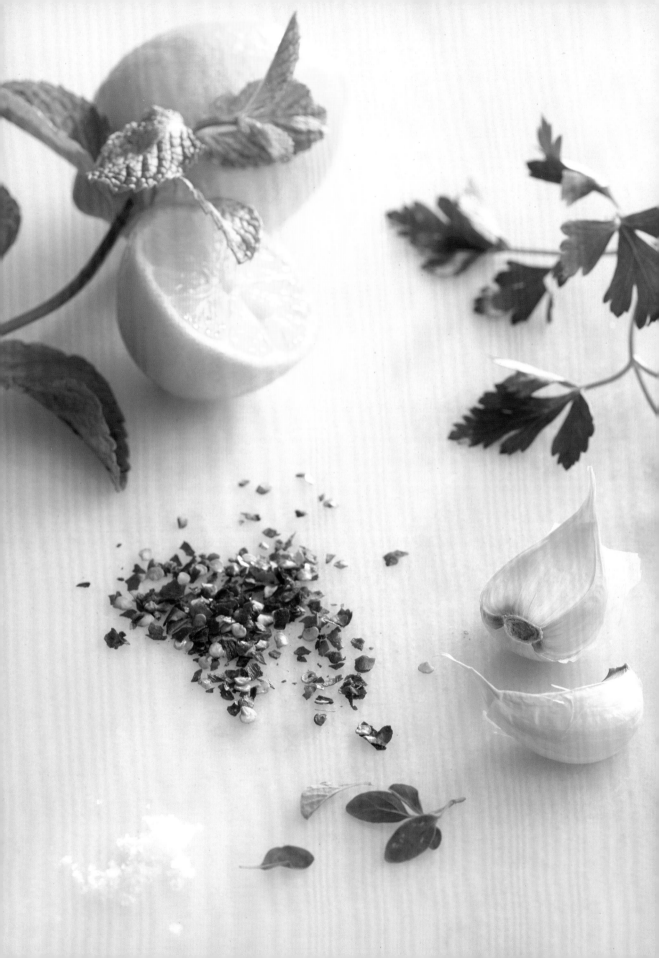

CHAPTER 8

Dollops

Dollops may seem like an afterthought, but they may well be the most important tool in your cooking arsenal. After all, neither man nor woman nor child can live on steamed broccoli alone. No matter how well intended one's desire to eat healthy, the fact is the taste buds have to stay enticed day in and day out to keep boredom from setting in (and boredom, as we all know, is the first step toward disconnecting from eating well). This is where dollops come in. From a taste perspective, these dollops are snazzy surprises, acting as delicious high notes on dishes ranging from fish to chicken, salads to soups, and more. Basil cashew cream, salsa verde, parsley pistou, minted chimichurri—more than a dozen, each ready to doll up any meal. The joy of these dollops is that, once made, they store well, and you'll never suffer from blah leftovers ever again. But there's more than just taste at work here. Many of the dollops contain healthy fats, which work to make brain-boosting vitamins and minerals more bioavailable. They also are full of interesting brain-enhancing chemicals in their own right. Take the walnut pesto dollop. Turns out the walnuts are full of melatonin, a sleep and relaxation aid. Who knew? Now you do.

BASIL CASHEW CREAM (PAGE 179)
Summer's Best Roasted Tomato and Red Bell Pepper Soup (page 53)

CILANTRO LIME VINAIGRETTE (PAGE 166)
Watercress, Purple Cabbage, and Edamame Salad with Toasted Sesame Seeds (page 75), Bejeweled Forbidden Rice Salad (page 144)

LEMON TAHINI DRESSING (PAGE 181)
Technicolor Slaw (page 73), Turkish Lamb Sliders (page 123), Falafel Mini Sliders (page 139)

MEYER LEMON BALSAMIC VINAIGRETTE (PAGE 172)
Arugula Salad with Roasted Cherries and Goat Cheese (page 72), or makes a great all-purpose dressing

MINTED CHIMICHURRI (PAGE 177)
Toasty Spiced Roasted Potatoes (page 101), Grilled Chicken with Za'atar (page 119), Baked Chicken with Minted Chimichurri (page 121), Rosemary and Thyme–Smothered Lamb Chops (page 127)

MY EVERYTHING DRIZZLE (PAGE 178)
Grilled Chicken with Za'atar (page 119), Mediterranean Roasted Chicken (page 122), all fish dishes

OLIVE AND SUN-DRIED TOMATO TAPENADE (PAGE 184)
Mediterranean Roasted Chicken (page 122), Triple Greens Frittata (page 141), Sweet Potato Hash (page 135)

ORANGE POMEGRANATE VINAIGRETTE (PAGE 171)
Orange Salad with Olives and Mint (page 81)

PARSLEY PISTOU (PAGE 175)
Sicilian Chicken Soup (page 60), Provençal Seafood Stew (page 61), Robust Chicken Soup (page 62), Mediterranean Roasted Chicken (page 122), Triple Greens Frittata (page 141), #SuperiorMoodSardines (page 138)

POMEGRANATE OLIVE MINT SALSA (PAGE 182)
Roasted Ginger Salmon with Pomegranate Olive Mint Salsa (page 114)

ROASTED TOMATO SAUCE (PAGE 167)
Quinoa Turkey Meatballs (page 116), fish, chicken, and vegetable dishes

SIGNORA FRANCINI'S SALSA VERDE (PAGE 174)
Italian White Bean Salad (page 79), Simple Shrimp Scampi (page 106), Baked Halibut with Tomato, Mint, and Fennel Vinaigrette (page 109), Quinoa Turkey Meatballs (page 116), Baked Chicken with Minted Chimichurri (page 121), Rosemary and Thyme–Smothered Lamb Chops (page 127)

TOASTED CUMIN CITRUS VINAIGRETTE (PAGE 170)
Lentil Salad with Roasted Beets and Toasted Cumin Citrus Vinaigrette (page 78), or use as a marinade for chicken or fish

TOMATO, MINT, AND FENNEL VINAIGRETTE (PAGE 173)
Baked Halibut with Tomato, Mint, and Fennel Vinaigrette (page 109), Black Cod Duvet (page 111), Grilled Chicken with Za'atar (page 119), Baked Chicken with Minted Chimichurri (page 121), Turkish Lamb Sliders (page 123)

TRICOLOR PEPPER SALSA (PAGE 168)
Summer's Best Roasted Tomato and Red Bell Pepper Soup (page 53), Baked Halibut with Tomato, Mint, and Fennel Vinaigrette (page 109), Quinoa Turkey Meatballs (page 116), Baked Chicken with Minted Chimichurri (page 121), Grilled Bison Burgers with Caramelized Onions and Crispy Shiitakes (page 125), with fish, chicken, or beef

WALNUT BASIL PESTO (PAGE 180)
Summer's Best Roasted Tomato and Red Bell Pepper Soup (page 53), Grilled Chicken with Za'atar (page 119)

YOGURT TAHINI RAITA (PAGE 185)
Moroccan Chickpea and Vegetable Soup (page 54), Turkish Lamb Sliders (page 123), Falafel Mini Sliders (page 139)

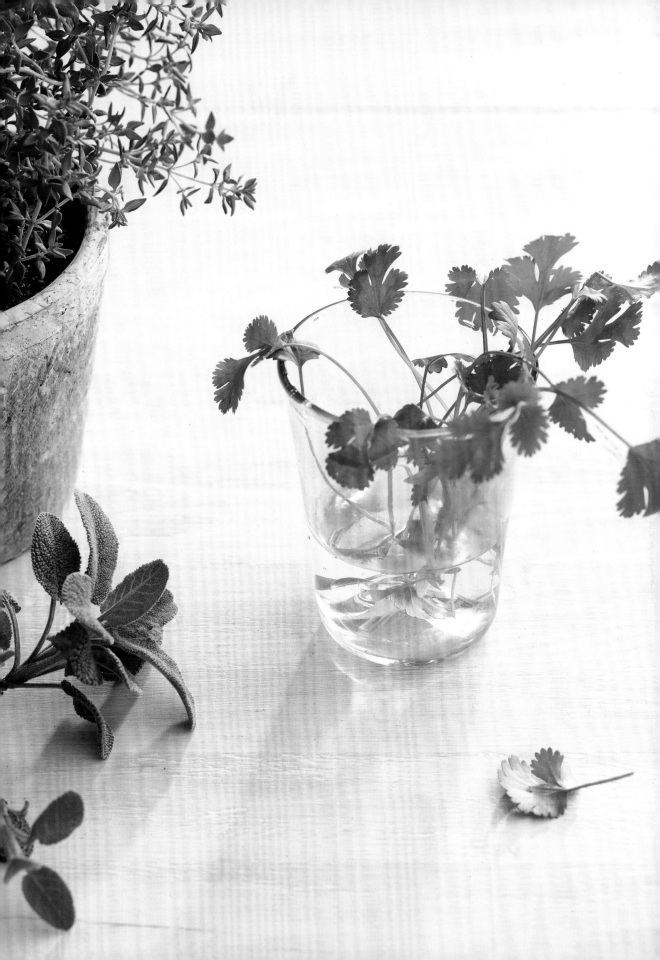

Cilantro Lime Vinaigrette

MAKES ABOUT ½ CUP • PREP TIME: 5 minutes • COOK TIME: Not applicable

Welcome, Little Mary Sunshine! This vinaigrette is light and bright, perfect for when you're looking for a dressing that allows a salad's ingredients to come through while adding just the right high note. Cilantro, with its high magnesium and iron content, offers a nice brain boost. In this book, I've paired it with the watercress and purple cabbage salad (page 75) and the forbidden rice salad (page 144).

½ cup cilantro

½ cup extra-virgin olive oil

1 teaspoon lime zest

3 tablespoons freshly squeezed lime juice

1 teaspoon grated fresh ginger

½ teaspoon Grade B maple syrup

½ teaspoon salt

Put all the ingredients in a small food processor and process about a minute, until smooth.

COOK'S NOTE: Cilantro tends to be a love-it-or-hate-it ingredient, and it turns out your opinion depends entirely on your DNA. Some folks have a gene that makes cilantro taste soapy, which makes it hard to become a fan of this healthful herb. If you're looking to replace cilantro in a recipe, try Italian flat-leaf parsley—it's a great power herb that will give you a similar nutritional wallop.

PER SERVING: Serving Size: 1 tablespoon; Calories: 183; Total Fat: 21 g (3 g saturated, 16.5 g monounsaturated); Carbohydrates: 0.7 g; Protein: 0.04 g; Fiber: 3 g; Sodium: 100 mg

STORAGE: Store in the refrigerator for up to 7 days.

Roasted Tomato Sauce

MAKES 4 CUPS • PREP TIME: 20 minutes • COOK TIME: 30 minutes

During the summer months, I take advantage of the abundance of tomatoes and put them in the oven to roast. The heavenly smells take me back to Italy, where I first learned how to make this version of tomato sauce. The tomatoes are gently pulsed in a food processor, which yields a lighter sauce. You don't have to reserve this sauce for pasta—dollop it on fish, vegetables, and meat dishes, including the quinoa meatballs on page 116.

Preheat the oven to 400°F.

Gently squeeze the tomatoes by hand to remove excess seeds, then put them in a bowl and toss with 1 tablespoon of the olive oil and $^1/_2$ teaspoon of salt. Place the tomatoes, cut side down, in a single layer on sheet pans and roast for 20 to 30 minutes, until the skins are just browning and the juices are bubbly. Let cool for 5 minutes, then lift off the skins with a fork.

Meanwhile, heat the remaining 1 tablespoon olive oil in a large saucepan, then add the onion and a pinch of salt and sauté until golden, about 5 minutes. Add the carrots, garlic, and $^1/_4$ teaspoon of salt and continue to sauté until the carrots become just tender, about 5 minutes.

Lift the tomatoes off the sheet pans and transfer to a food processor, then pour in any pan juices. Add the carrot mixture and the basil and pulse until pureed but still a little chunky. Transfer back into the saucepan and stir in $^1/_4$ teaspoon of salt. Taste. Tomatoes can sometimes be acidic, so you may want to add a pinch of sweetener and another pinch of salt.

VARIATION: If fresh tomatoes aren't available, you can substitute two 28-ounce cans of plum tomatoes.

PER SERVING: Serving Size: 1 tablespoon; Calories: 120; Total Fat: 5.4 g (0.8 g saturated, 3.5 g monounsaturated); Carbohydrates: 17 g; Protein: 4 g; Fiber: 5 g; Sodium: 230 mg

STORAGE: Store in an airtight container in the refrigerator for 5 days or in thefreezer for 3 months.

4 pounds Roma or San Marzano tomatoes, halved

2 tablespoons extra-virgin olive oil

Sea salt

1 onion, diced small

2 carrots, scrubbed and diced small

2 cloves garlic, chopped

2 cups loosely packed fresh basil leaves, chopped

Tricolor Pepper Salsa

MAKES 1¹/₄ CUPS • PREP TIME: 10 minutes • COOK TIME: Not applicable

Sometimes food needs a little love, a little bling to provide some zing to what might otherwise be a bland taste. That's where this salsa provides both some eye candy and a bright, fresh, crunchy taste. This is a summer shot of goodness, bringing together onions, cherry tomatoes, yellow and red bell peppers, basil, olive oil, and lemon zest. It goes great with halibut or grilled chicken or meat, and it's also a super dipping salsa.

¹/₄ cup finely diced red onion

6 cherry tomatoes, halved

2 tablespoons finely diced red bell pepper

2 tablespoons finely diced yellow bell pepper

3 tablespoons extra-virgin olive oil

¹/₄ cup chopped fresh basil or mint

1¹/₂ tablespoons freshly squeezed lemon juice

¹/₂ teaspoon lemon zest

1 tablespoon chopped fresh parsley

¹/₄ teaspoon sea salt

¹/₄ teaspoon freshly ground black pepper

In a large bowl, combine all the ingredients. Cover and refrigerate until ready to use.

PER SERVING: Serving Size: 1 tablespoon; Calories: 16; Total Fat: 1.6 g (0.2 g saturated, 1.2 g monounsaturated); Carbohydrates: 0.7 g; Protein: 0.1 g; Fiber: 0.2 g; Sodium: 12 mg

STORAGE: Refrigerate in an airtight container for 1 day.

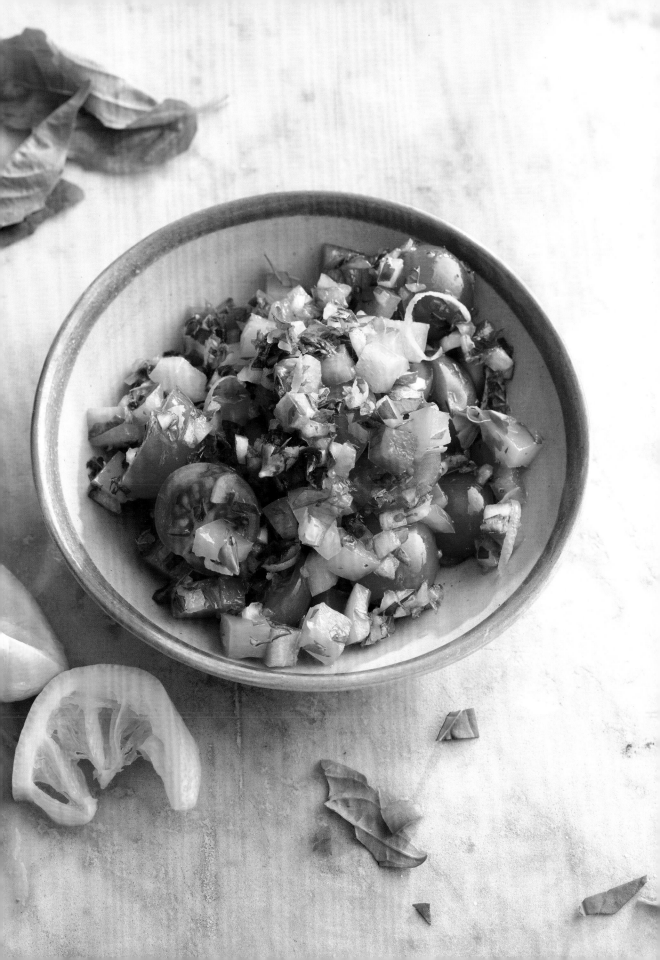

Toasted Cumin Citrus Vinaigrette

I come by making salad dressing honestly, as my dad was in the food manufacturing business. Many a day I'd come to my dad's office with my latest vinaigrette concoction in a yogurt cup and take it to the lab, where I learned to measure ingredients precisely so we could reproduce the taste in my little yogurt cup when it was scaled up to a two-hundred-gallon drum (talk about the importance of learning how to write down a repeatable recipe!). This airtight dressing is easy to prepare and delicious. It's a fantastic go-to salad dressing, and works great with fish, chicken, or, in this book, the Lentil Salad with Roasted Beets (page 78).

2 oranges, zested

1/2 cup freshly squeezed orange juice

2 tablespoons freshly squeezed lemon juice

2 teaspoons cumin seeds, toasted

1/4 teaspoon sea salt

1/4 teaspoon freshly ground black pepper

1/2 cup extra-virgin olive oil

Put the orange zest, orange juice, lemon juice, cumin seeds, salt, and pepper in a small bowl and stir to combine. Slowly pour in the olive oil, whisking all the while, and continue whisking until smooth. Transfer to a small container with a fitted lid and shake well.

COOK'S NOTE: This vinaigrette masquerades as either a salad dressing or an excellent marinade for chicken or fish.

PER SERVING: Serving Size: 1 tablespoon; Calories: 130; Total Fat: 14 g (2 g saturated, 11 g monounsaturated); Carbohydrates: 2.2 g; Protein: 0.23 g; Fiber: 0.17 g; Sodium: 51 mg

STORAGE: Store in an airtight container in the refrigerator for up to 5 days.

Orange Pomegranate Vinaigrette

MAKES ABOUT ¹/₂ CUP • PREP TIME: 5 minutes • COOK TIME: Not applicable

A little song, a little dance . . . this is sweet-and-sour doing a delightful tango on the taste buds, with the intense tartness of the pomegranate molasses magnificently mollified by the orange's mellow sweetness. This vinaigrette partners delightfully with just about any salad that happens to sashay its way.

Put the orange juice, lemon zest, lemon juice, pomegranate molasses, salt, and pepper in a small bowl and stir to combine. Slowly pour in the olive oil, whisking all the while, and continue whisking until smooth. Transfer to a small container with a fitted lid and shake well.

COOK'S NOTE: You can substitute balsamic vinegar if you don't have pomegranate molasses.

PER SERVING: Serving Size: 1 tablespoon; Calories: 136; Total Fat: 14 g (1 g saturated, 11 g monounsaturated); Carbohydrates: 4 g; Protein: 0.10 g; Fiber: 0.12 g; Sodium: 200 mg

STORAGE: Store in an airtight container in the refrigerator for up to 5 days.

1 tablespoon freshly squeezed orange juice

1 teaspoon grated lemon zest

2 tablespoons freshly squeezed lemon juice

1 tablespoon pomegranate molasses

¹/₂ teaspoon sea salt

¹/₂ teaspoon freshly ground black pepper

¹/₄ cup extra-virgin olive oil

Meyer Lemon Balsamic Vinaigrette

MAKES ABOUT ¹/₂ CUP • PREP TIME: 5 minutes • COOK TIME: Not applicable

Another good all-purpose salad dressing that comes together quickly and lasts for a week in the fridge. I love Meyer lemons because, relative to other lemons, they're quite sweet. If you don't have a few Meyers hanging around, use a combination of regular lemon juice and orange juice.

2 tablespoons balsamic vinegar

¹/₂ teaspoon grated lemon zest

2 tablespoons freshly squeezed Meyer lemon juice

¹/₂ teaspoon sea salt

¹/₂ teaspoon freshly ground black pepper

¹/₄ cup extra-virgin olive oil

1 tablespoon minced shallot (optional)

Put the balsamic vinegar, lemon zest, lemon juice, salt, and pepper in a small bowl and stir to combine. Slowly pour in the olive oil, whisking all the while, and continue whisking until smooth. Transfer to a small container with a fitted lid and shake well.

COOK'S NOTES: Add the salt with the acid but *prior* to adding the oil. The reason? The acid breaks down the salt, allowing it to do its job as a flavor carrier.

The Meyer lemon is milder and sweeter tasting than most store-bought lemons. If you don't have Meyer lemons, use 2 tablespoons of lemon juice combined with 2 tablespoons of freshly squeezed tangerine or orange juice. As for the zest, regular lemon zest is an acceptable substitute.

PER SERVING: Serving Size: 1 tablespoon; Calories: 129; Total Fat: 14 g (2 g saturated, 11 g monounsaturated); Carbohydrates: 2 g; Protein: 0.12 g; Fiber: 0.2 g; Sodium: 203 mg

STORAGE: Store in an airtight container in the refrigerator for up to 5 days.

Tomato, Mint, and Fennel Vinaigrette

MAKES ABOUT ³/4 CUP · PREP TIME: 10 minutes · COOK TIME: Not applicable

I have a tendency to get close to my creations. Maybe a little too close. I served this vinaigrette recently, and it was a big hit. The best part, thought I, was I had plenty left over to experiment with for the rest of the week. That was before my husband did the dishes and accidentally threw out the batch. You would have thought it was his wedding ring that he'd flushed down the drain. I went off like a madwoman—all I could think of, through my red haze, was how Italian cooks shout "senza rispetto!" when they feel dissed—and I was so worked up I actually gave myself a time-out. A few minutes later there was a knock at the door. Poor Gregg was standing there, sheepishly apologizing (he hadn't really done anything wrong, I was just being a prima donna). He felt so bad, he promised he'd make me another batch. Ah, it's tough to be the cook . . .

Put the lemon juice, mustard, salt, pepper, fennel seeds, and shallot in a small bowl and whisk to combine. Slowly pour in the olive oil, whisking all the while, and continue whisking until smooth. Transfer to a small container with a fitted lid and shake well. Then, add the olives, tomatoes, and mint and gently stir to combine.

VARIATIONS: You can substitute cumin seeds for the fennel seeds. If tomatoes are not in season, use a small jar of roasted red peppers instead.

COOK'S NOTE: You can crush the fennel seeds in a mortar and pestle or in a small bowl with the back of a spoon.

PER SERVING: Serving Size: 1 tablespoon; Calories: 110; Total Fat: 11 g (1.6 g saturated, 9 g monounsaturated); Carbohydrates: 2.6 g; Protein: 0.5 g; Fiber: 0.6 g; Sodium: 268 mg

STORAGE: Store in an airtight container in the refrigerator for up to 5 days.

3 tablespoons freshly squeezed lemon juice

1 teaspoon Dijon mustard

¹/2 teaspoon sea salt

¹/8 teaspoon freshly ground black pepper

1¹/2 teaspoons fennel seeds, toasted and crushed (see Cook's Note)

1 tablespoon minced shallot

¹/4 cup extra-virgin olive oil

12 kalamata olives, chopped

¹/2 cup chopped tomatoes

2 tablespoons finely chopped fresh mint

Signora Francini's Salsa Verde

MAKES ABOUT 1 CUP • PREP TIME: 5 minutes • COOK TIME: Not applicable

Can a minute—and a sauce—change your life? I'm here to tell you they can. I was wandering through Florence about twenty years ago, before I was a cook, wondering where life was going to take me. I had signed up for a cooking class—my first—but was given the wrong location. I showed up an hour *early* (and believe me, I'm not early for anything). I was literally a minute away from walking out of the classroom when the teacher walked in, pointed at me, and said in Italian, "Walk this way." She led me into her kitchen, where the other students had already gathered, and began making basic Italian sauces. The scene—the kitchen was right over a bustling an Italian market—and the aromas soon began to fill my head, and as I chopped away at the parsley for the salsa verde, I was embraced with that rarest of feelings, of being exactly in the right place at the right time doing the right thing. The teacher, Judy Witts Francini, not only lit my fire for cooking, she *was* the fire, going on to become one of my closest culinary friends. She set the path, and I followed. So, yes, life can change in a minute. Mine certainly did, and I'm forever grateful.

2 cups coarsely chopped fresh parsley leaves

1/2 teaspoon sea salt

4 anchovy fillets, rinsed

1/4 cup freshly squeezed lemon juice

4 teaspoons capers, rinsed

1/4 teaspoon freshly ground pepper

1/2 cup extra-virgin olive oil

Put all the ingredients except the olive oil in a food processor and blend for about a minute, until finely chopped. With the food processor running, drizzle in the olive oil and process until the sauce is smooth.

PER SERVING: Serving Size: 1 tablespoon; Calories: 133; Total Fat: 14 g (2 g saturated, 11 g monounsaturated); Carbohydrates: 1.8 g; Protein: 1 g; Fiber: 0.65 g; Sodium: 126 mg

STORAGE: Store in the refrigerator for up to 7 days.

Parsley Pistou

MAKES ABOUT $^3/_4$ CUP • PREP TIME: 5 minutes • COOK TIME: Not applicable

Pistou might sound strange (or remind you of a six-shooter), but it's just pesto minus the nuts. For me, the right pistou is aromatherapy, blowing out all the cobwebs. Think about how your brain responded the last time you waved some fresh mint under your nose; suddenly your senses were on full, friendly, alert. Basil is from the same family as mint, and combined with another clean, fresh herb in parsley, creates a drizzle that dazzles. It boosts the taste altimeter through the roof when spooned over fish, chicken, or veggies.

Combine the parsley, basil, lemon juice, garlic, $^1/_4$ teaspoon of salt, and olive oil in a food processor and process until well blended. For a thinner drizzle, add a tablespoon of water and briefly process again. Taste; you may want to add a pinch of salt.

1 cup tightly packed fresh parsley leaves

$^1/_2$ cup tightly packed fresh basil leaves

2 tablespoons freshly squeezed lemon juice

2 teaspoons garlic

Sea salt

$^1/_4$ cup extra-virgin olive oil

PER SERVING: Serving Size: 1 tablespoon; Calories: 44; Total Fat: 4.7 g (0.7 g saturated, 3.7 g monounsaturated); Carbohydrates: 0.8 g; Protein: 0.3 g; Fiber: 0.27 g; Sodium: 37 mg

STORAGE: Store in an airtight container in the refrigerator for up to 5 days.

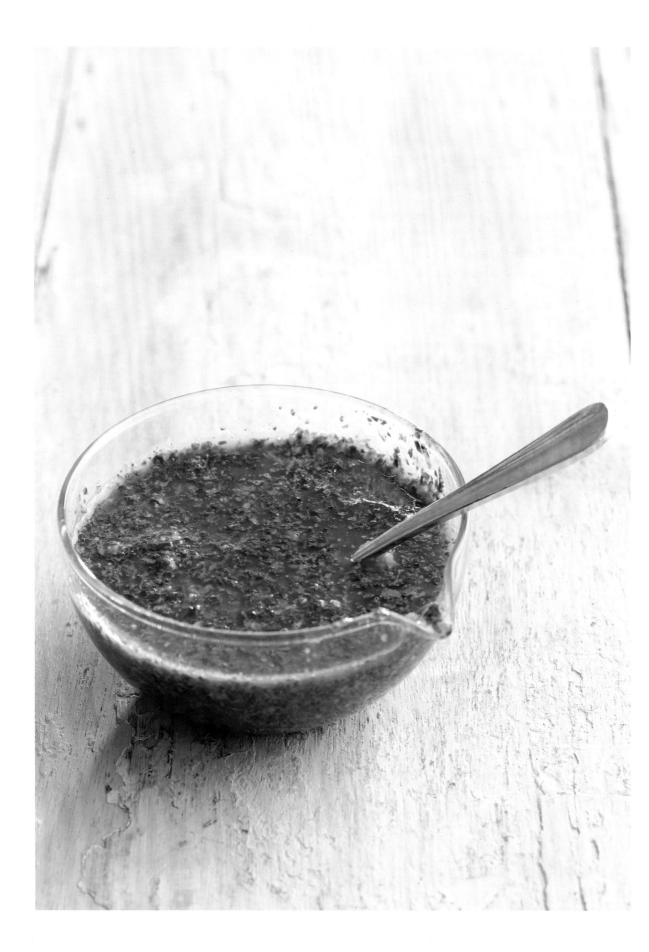

Minted Chimichurri

Chimichurri is to South America as salsa verde is to Italy. Or maybe it's simpler to call it Argentinian barbecue sauce. My version combines parsley, garlic, red pepper flakes, olive oil, lemon juice, and the kicker, mint. The scent of mint has been shown to increase alertness, and the taste is perfect for waking up chicken and other meats. As the Argentines might say, this is a chimichuri that adds *destello* (sparkle) to a dish.

Add all the ingredients to a blender or food processor and process until all the ingredients are well combined.

PER SERVING: Serving Size: 1 tablespoon; Calories: 88.5; Total Fat: 9.5 g (1.3 g saturated, 7.3 g monounsaturated); Carbohydrates: 1.3 g; Protein: 0.22 g; Fiber: 0.28 g; Sodium: 52 mg

STORAGE: Store in an airtight container in the refrigerator for up to 5 days

3/4 cup tightly packed fresh mint

3/4 cup tightly packed flat-leaf parsley

1/3 cup fresh oregano, or 2 tablespoons dried

4 cloves garlic, minced

1/2 teaspoon red pepper flakes

1/2 teaspoon sea salt

2 teaspoons lemon zest

1/3 cup freshly squeezed lemon juice

2/3 cup extra-virgin olive oil

My Everything Drizzle

MAKES ABOUT ¹/₂ CUP • PREP TIME: 5 minutes • COOK TIME: Not applicable

This is the dollop that's always front and center in my refrigerator. The combination of fresh parsley and mint, blended with lemon, olive oil, and sea salt is a perfect drizzle to amp up the yum for chicken, lamb, fish, or vegetables. I've been known to scrape the jar, just to capture the last few drops. Parsley gets a brain boost from the phytochemical quercetin, which helps protect brain cells from free radical damage, while mint helps with focus and concentration.

Combine the parsley, mint, lemon juice, ¹/₈ teaspoon of salt, syrup, and oil in a food processor and process until well blended. For a thinner drizzle, add a tablespoon of water and briefly process again. Taste; you may want to add a pinch of salt.

COOK'S NOTE: To quickly remove stems from parsley or cilantro, hold a clean, dry bunch of the herbs in your noncutting hand, angling them downward at 45 degrees, with the top of the bunch touching the cutting board. Scrape down along the stems with a chef's knife, using short strokes, to separate the leaves from the stems.

PER SERVING: Serving Size: 1 tablespoon; Calories: 63; Total Fat: 7 g (1 g saturated, 5.5 g monounsaturated); Carbohydrates: 0.5 g; Protein: 0 g; Fiber: 0 g; Sodium: 27 mg

STORAGE: Store in an airtight container in the refrigerator for up to 5 days.

¹/₂ cup tightly packed fresh parsley leaves

2 tablespoons tightly packed fresh mint leaves

1 tablespoon freshly squeezed lemon juice

Sea salt

¹/₄ teaspoon Grade B maple syrup

¹/₄ cup extra-virgin olive oil

Basil Cashew Cream

MAKES ABOUT 2 CUPS · PREP TIME: 5 minutes · COOK TIME: Not applicable

Oh, do I love working with cashews. They're the perfect creamy nut, so much so that used as a dollop you'll swear you're eating actual cream. But you're not (heh-heh); you're eating something that's full of brain-boosting minerals. I use cashew cream with Summer's Best Roasted Tomato and Red Bell Pepper Soup (page 53), but it's also delightful drizzled over veggies or grains. I call cashew cream The Great Pretender, but there's nothing fake about the taste; you'll devour it.

Grind the cashews in a mini food processor or nut grinder to give them a head start in the blender (if you have a Vitamix or other heavy duty blender, you can skip this step). Put the water in the blender, then add the lemon juice, salt, and cashews and blend until creamy-smooth. Add the basil and blend again until beautifully creamy and light green. This takes several minutes, but your taste buds will reap the rewards of your patience.

1 cup cashews

1 cup water

1 teaspoons freshly squeezed lemon juice

$1/4$ teaspoon sea salt

$1/2$ cup loosely packed fresh basil leaves

PER SERVING: Serving Size: 1 tablespoon; Calories: 49; Total Fat: 4 g (1 g saturated, 2 g monounsaturated); Carbohydrates: 3 g; Protein: 2 g; Fiber: 0.31 g; Sodium: 26 mg

STORAGE: Store in an airtight container in the refrigerator for up to 5 days or in the freezer for up to 2 months.

Walnut Basil Pesto

MAKES ABOUT ²/₃ CUP · PREP TIME: 5 minutes · COOK TIME: Not applicable

Just like *A Star Is Born*, sometimes you have to remake a classic with a more modern twist. Here, I take pesto and use walnuts instead of pine nuts, but it's still simple to put together, as basil, walnuts, olive oil, sea salt, and water all go right into the food processor. It's a wonderful all-purpose pesto that, as I like to say, is great to have in your back pocket anytime you're making lamb, chicken, fish, or tomato soup.

Place the walnuts in a food processor and pulse 5 times, until they are broken into small pieces. Add basil, olive oil, 1 tablespoon of lemon juice, maple syrup, and ¹/₄ teaspoon of salt, and process until well blended. For a thinner pesto, add the water and briefly process again. Taste; you may want to add an additional squeeze of lemon juice or a pinch of salt.

PER SERVING: Serving Size: 1 tablespoon; Calories: 98; Total Fat: 11 g (1 g saturated, 6 g monounsaturated); Carbohydrates: 1 g; Protein: 1 g; Fiber: 0.5 g; Sodium: 38 mg

STORAGE: Store in an airtight container in the refrigerator for up to 5 days or in the freezer for up to 2 months.

¹/₂ cup walnuts, toasted

1 cup tightly packed basil leaves

¹/₃ cup extra-virgin olive oil

Freshly squeezed Meyer lemon juice

¹/₂ teaspoon Grade B maple syrup

Sea salt

Lemon Tahini Dressing

MAKES ABOUT 1/4 CUP • PREP TIME: 5 minutes • COOK TIME: Not applicable

"Tahini" sounds exotic, kind of like Tahiti, but if you can get past the name it's one of the simplest ingredients in this most basic—but delicious, of course—of dressings. Tahini is a sesame paste, available in any supermarket, and a major player in hummus. It's so easy to work with that this whole dressing comes together with nothing more than a fork, a little warm water, some lemon juice, and couple of spices. I use tahini for the taste, but your body will love it for its high healthy fat and mineral content including zinc, which is important in learning and brain development.

Put the tahini, lemon juice, salt, maple syrup, cumin, cinnamon, and cayenne in a small bowl and mix with a spoon into a smooth paste. Slowly pour in the warm water, whisking all the while and continue whisking until you've achieved a thick but pourable dressing. If more water is needed, add a teaspoon at a time. Season with pepper if desired.

PER SERVING: Serving Size: 1 tablespoon; Calories: 197; Total Fat: 18 g (2.5 g saturated, 0 g monounsaturated); Carbohydrates: 5 g; Protein: 8 g; Fiber: 1.2 g; Sodium: 211 mg

STORAGE: Store in the refrigerator for about a week. The dressing thickens as it sits, so you may need to add more water to thin.

1/4 cup tahini

2 tablespoons freshly squeezed lemon juice

1/4 teaspoon sea salt

1/4 teaspoon maple syrup

1/4 teaspoon ground cumin

1/8 teaspoon ground cinnamon

Pinch of cayenne pepper

2 tablespoons warm water, plus more as needed

Freshly ground black pepper (optional)

Pomegranate Olive Mint Salsa

MAKES ABOUT 2¹/₂ CUPS • PREP TIME: 15 minutes • COOK TIME: Not applicable •

Painting, like cooking, is all about getting into a zone, which is probably why I like doing both. They're complementary in another way; I'm visually driven, and when I'm working on a painting—as I was this past summer—I'm drawn to foods that create a color sensation on the plate. Don't ask me why—maybe there's something about color that impacts taste—but foods that blend well visually also taste fantastic together. I know that not many people would put pomegranate seeds together with olives and fennel, but you gotta trust me on this one; it's not only a dance party for the mouth, but your eyes will widen at how good it looks.

1 cup finely chopped flat-leaf parsley

¹/₄ cup finely chopped mint

¹/₂ cup kalamata or green olives, chopped

¹/₂ cup finely chopped fennel

¹/₄ cup pomegranate seeds

¹/₄ cup chopped walnuts, toasted

2 scallions, minced

1 tablespoon extra-virgin olive oil

Freshly squeezed lemon juice

¹/₂ teaspoon freshly ground black pepper

Sea salt

Put the parsley, mint, olives, fennel, pomegranate seeds, walnuts, scallions, olive oil, 2 teaspoons of lemon juice, black pepper, and a pinch of salt in a bowl and stir gently to combine. For optimal flavor, cover and let sit at room temperature for 15 minutes before serving. Taste; you may want to add another squeeze of lemon or a pinch of salt.

PER SERVING: Serving Size: ¹/₄ cup; Calories: 33; Total Fat: 3 g (0.30 g saturated, 1.6 g monounsaturated); Carbohydrates: 1.5 g; Protein: 0.5 g; Fiber: 0.4 g; Sodium: 97 mg

STORAGE: Store in an airtight container in the refrigerator for up to 4 days.

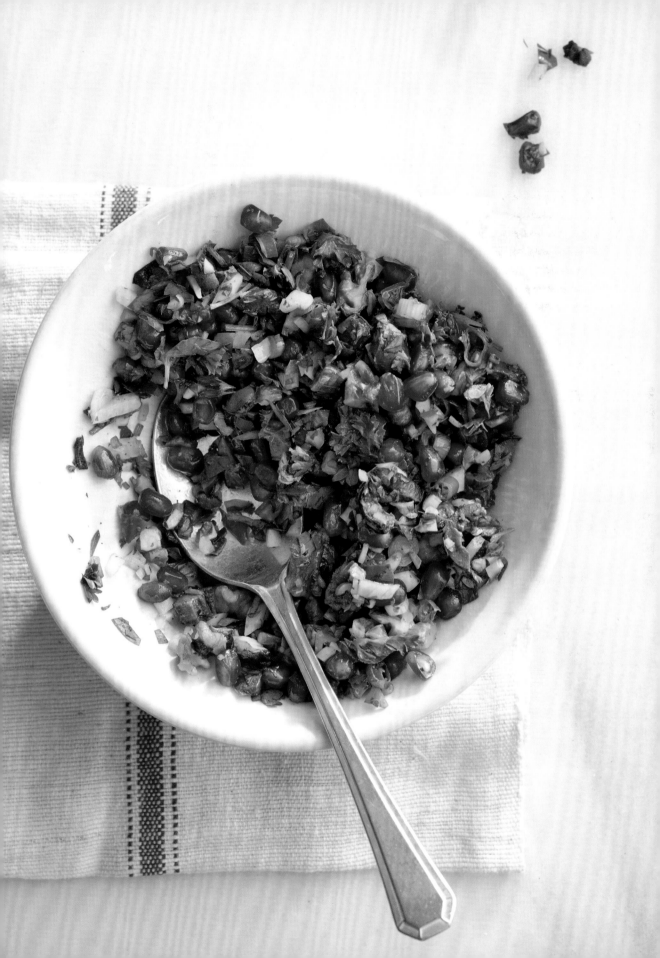

Olive and Sun-Dried Tomato Tapenade

MAKES ²/3 CUP • PREP TIME: 5 minutes • COOK TIME: Not applicable

Once upon a time, I was a chef at a restaurant with a crew who could only be described as a bunch of pirates in training. Surf bums, ne'er-do-wells, rapscallions . . . and little old me, with only my East Coast attitude to keep them all in line. They never did understand why I took things like tapenades—an afterthought in many kitchens—so seriously. They called me the Condiment Queen (well, I'm sure they called me lots of other things, but not to my face). Then came the night a top chef ate at our shop. He gave the waiter a message: "Tell the chef that was the most well-appointed tapenade I've ever eaten." The message was delivered, and every eye in the kitchen was suddenly on me. I didn't even raise my head, but I did speak. "And that," I told my crew in a quiet voice, "is why I pay attention to my tapenade."

¹/2 cup tightly packed fresh basil leaves

¹/4 cup niçoise olives, pitted and coarsely chopped

12 kalamata olives, pitted and coarsely chopped

¹/4 cup sun-dried tomatoes in olive oil, coarsely chopped

1 heaping teaspoon capers, rinsed

1 teaspoon chopped garlic

Pinch of red pepper flakes

1 teaspoon lemon zest

Freshly squeezed Meyer lemon juice

¹/3 cup extra-virgin olive oil

Sea salt

Put the basil, olives, tomatoes, capers, garlic, red pepper flakes, lemon zest, 1 tablespoon lemon juice, and olive oil in a food processor and process until well blended. Taste; you may want to add an additional squeeze of lemon juice or a pinch of salt.

PER SERVING: Serving Size: 1 tablespoon; Calories: 91; Total Fat: 9.6 g (1.3 g saturated, 7.4 g monounsaturated); Carbohydrates: 1.7 g; Protein: 0.4 g; Fiber: 0.3 g; Sodium: 153 mg

STORAGE: Store in an airtight container in the refrigerator for up to 5 days or in the freezer for up to 2 months

Yogurt Tahini Raita

MAKES ABOUT 1 CUP • PREP TIME: 10 minutes • COOK TIME: Not applicable

Part of the fun of cooking is using words that taste good as they come off the tongue. "Tahini" and "raita" fit the bill, but here's the secret: they're nothing fancy, just delicious. Tahini is a ground sesame seed paste used in Middle Eastern cooking, while raita is a yogurt-based sauce that contains tons of antioxidant and anti-inflammatory rich herbs and spices. The yogurt is full of probiotics, which promotes good gut and brain health.

½ cup plain organic Greek yogurt

¼ cup tahini

1 teaspoon lemon zest

2 to 3 tablespoons freshly squeezed lemon juice

2 pinches of sea salt

Pinch of cayenne pepper

⅛ teaspoon Grade B maple syrup

1 to 2 tablespoons water, as needed for consistency

⅓ cup peeled, seeded, and minced cucumber

2 tablespoons finely chopped fresh mint

In a bowl, whisk together the yogurt, tahini, zest, lemon juice, salt, cayenne, and maple syrup. Stir in enough water to achieve a spoonable consistency. Fold in the cucumber and mint.

PER SERVING: Serving Size: 1 tablespoon; Calories: 69; Total Fat: 6 g (1.8 g saturated, 0 g monounsaturated); Carbohydrates: 2 g; Protein: 3 g; Fiber: 0.4 g; Sodium: 57 mg

STORAGE: Store in an airtight container in the refrigerator for up to 5 days.

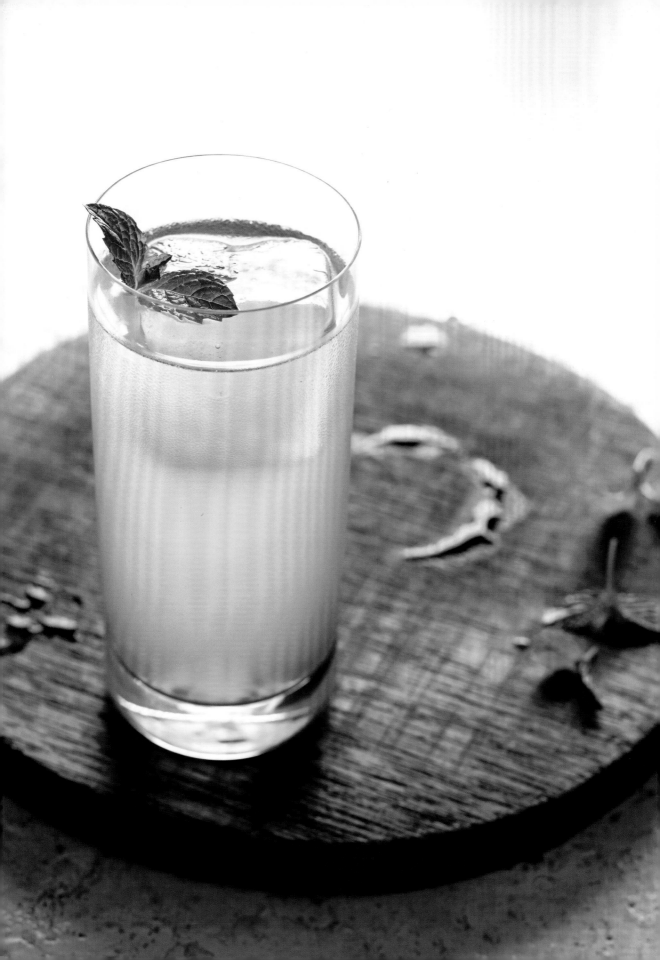

CHAPTER 9

Tonics and Elixirs

A little fluid can go a long way in keeping the brain happy. Consider that even a 1 to 2 percent loss of fluid levels in the brain has been linked to a host of mental impairments, including attention deficit, slower processing, and poorer short-term memory retention. It's readily apparent that hydration is the key to neuronal nirvana—neurons actually *shrink* when they don't get enough fluid. What's wonderful about these tonics and elixirs is that they hydrate in the best way possible—by introducing both nutrients and fiber that slows down water so it doesn't just pass through the body, but rather stops and stays awhile to get absorbed in the gut. Just as important, you can choose a drink based on whether you need to relax (chamomile lavender tea lemonade), recharge (ginger-mint infused water), or just blow away mental fatigue (pomegranate mock mojito). There are fifteen drinks in all, and all contribute in some way—besides hydration—to brain health, offering antioxidants and anti-inflammatory benefits. The tastes are unique and unforgettable, and are a wonderful antidote for people who want to get fluids but are flat-out bored by the taste of straight water. These tonics and elixirs are everything you could want in a glass, guaranteed to gloriously suffuse your mind and mouth with liquid ambrosia.

Chamomile Lavender Lemonade

MAKES 1 QUART · PREP TIME: 5 minutes · COOK TIME: 5 minutes

Some drinks are meant to be savored—no grab-and-go, but sit, sip, and feel the day's tension melt away. Chamomile and lavender will do that to you; aromatherapists have long used essential oil of lavender as a calmative. Here, mixed with chamomile and lemon juice to make it a soothing lemonade, it's a major stress buster.

4 bags Traditional Medicinals chamomile with lavender and lemon balm tea

2 tablespoons honey

1/2 cup freshly squeezed lemon juice

Bring 4 cups of water to a boil; add the tea bags and let steep for 5 minutes. Add honey and stir to dissolve, then stir in the lemon juice. Serve warm or on ice.

COOK'S NOTE: Any combination of chamomile and lavender or chamomile and ginger tea bags will work.

PER SERVING: Serving Size: 1 cup; Calories: 41; Total Fat: 0 g (0 g saturated, 0 g monounsaturated); Carbohydrates: 11 g; Protein: 0 g; Fiber: 0 g; Sodium: 5.5 mg

STORAGE: Store in an airtight container in the refrigerator for up to 4 days.

Blackberry and Sage H$_2$O

MAKES 2 QUARTS • PREP TIME: 5 minutes • COOK TIME: Not applicable

You can always tell when a fad has taken off when you start seeing it showing up in refrigerators in gas station quickie-marts. So it is with "infused water," which, commercially bought, is about as exciting (and nutritionally helpful) as drinking Kool-Aid. That's not the case here. Waters infused with the right ingredients are tonics for the senses, and this water looks like wine and tastes like heaven. Sage, as the name implies, has been tied to raising IQs. Sage also softens the usually sour nature of blackberry, making the water taste, in my assistant Jen's words, "pillowy." She assures me it's a comfortable pillow, one where you'd love to rest your head.

Put all the ingredients in a pitcher and let sit for at least 30 minutes. Strain when you're satisfied with the flavor, or let it keep infusing until you've drunk it up. The longer it sits, the more flavor will be infused.

8 cups filtered water

4 large sage leaves, rubbed between your hands

1^1/$_4$ cups fresh or frozen blackberries

COOK'S NOTE: This is the perfect elixir to have in a glass pitcher on your desk. It's beautiful to the eye and boosting to the brain. If you use frozen berries, they'll act as ice cubes.

PER SERVING: Serving Size: 1 cup; Calories: 10; Total Fat: 0 g (0 g saturated, 0 g monounsaturated); Carbohydrates: 2 g; Protein: 0.5 g; Fiber: 1 g; Sodium: 5.5 mg

STORAGE: Store in an airtight container in the refrigerator for up to 4 days.

Pomegranate Mock Mojito

The wonderful thing about cooking is that we can borrow from everywhere. Take bartending: one of their favorite tools is the muddler, which, as the name implies, muddles (or crushes) ingredients to release flavors that go into the drink. And so it is here, with mint being the ingredient to be muddled. Now, you and I don't have muddlers (unless you happen to be a mixologist), but you can use a mortar and pestle or the back of a wooden spoon to break down the mint and release the essential oils that go into this mojito. Mixed with antioxidant-rich pomegranate juice, lime juice, and *pellegrino* (Italian for "seltzer"), it tastes anything but muddled; it's a straight shot of joy juice to the brain.

1/2 cup freshly squeezed lime juice

1/2 cup pomegranate juice

2 teaspoons honey, optional

24 sprigs spearmint or peppermint

1 cup seltzer water

Ice

Put the lime juice, pomegranate juice, and honey into a large measuring cup and stir to combine. Add the mint leaves and crush with a wooden spoon against the side of the cup. Add the mineral water and stir. Pour into two glasses filled with ice and serve immediately.

VARIATIONS: Use cranberry juice or blueberry juice in place of the pomegranate juice.

PER SERVING: Serving Size: 1 cup; Calories: 37; Total Fat: .5 g (0 g saturated, 0 g monounsaturated); Carbohydrates: 10 g; Protein: 1 g; Fiber: 1 g; Sodium: 2 mg

STORAGE: Not applicable

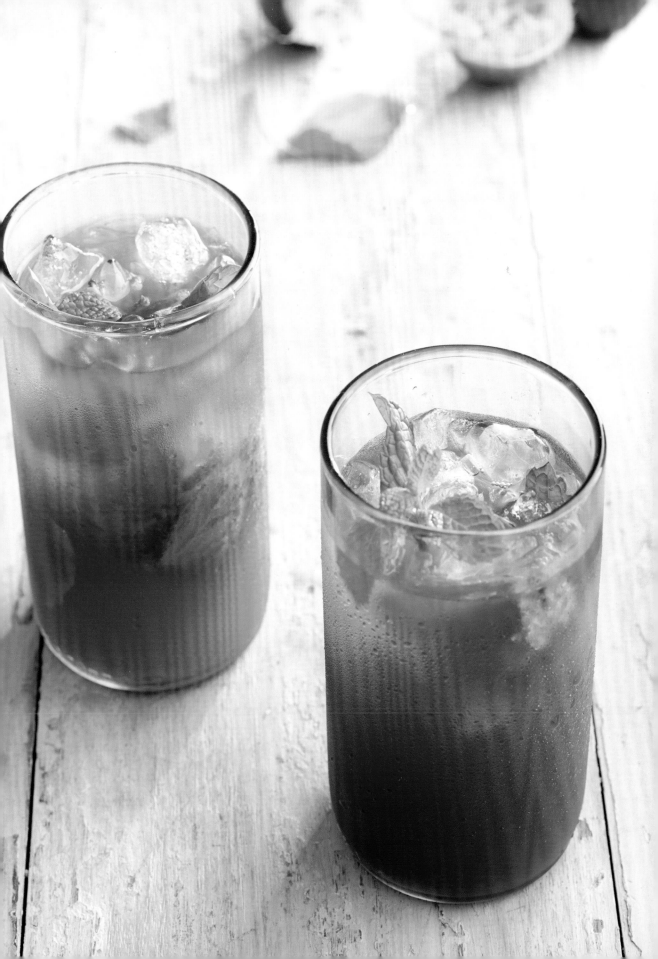

Ginger Mint Tea

MAKES 1 QUART · PREP TIME: 5 minutes · COOK TIME: 15 minutes.

It's funny the memories that flash through your mind when you cook. When I was a kid, my mom's solution for clogged sinuses was steam. So there I'd sit, hovering over a hot pot of water set in the sink, with a large towel draped over my head. It looked funny, but it worked (for a few minutes, anyway). Well, this concoction puts me in the way-back machine; as the twelve sprigs of peppermint come to a boil, the steaming aroma clears out my sinuses but good. The ginger just adds to the fresh headiness of the brew: one sip will blow out all the cobwebs.

8 cups filtered water

1 cup sliced unpeeled fresh ginger

1 cup loosely packed fresh peppermint or spearmint leaves

Put all the ingredients in a pot over high heat. Cover and bring to a boil; uncover, and lower the heat to simmer for 15 minutes. Strain when you're satisfied with the flavor, or let it keep infusing until you've drunk it all. Drink warm or iced.

COOK'S NOTE: Peppermint is a stronger and more assertive mint, which is great for tea. Spearmint is milder and sweeter and is often used in cooking. Either mint will work in this brew.

PER SERVING: Serving Size: 1 cup; Calories: 0; Total Fat: 0 g (0 g saturated, 0 g monounsaturated); Carbohydrates: 5 g; Protein: 1 g; Fiber: 0 g; Sodium: 15 mg

STORAGE: Store in an airtight container in the refrigerator for up to 4 days.

Triple Citrus Cooler

MAKES 2 SERVINGS · PREP TIME: 5 minutes · COOK TIME: 25 minutes

When I want to go from "wow" to "YOWZA!" with a drink, I boil it down into a syrup. This one's made with grapefruit, lemon, and orange. And sometimes inspiration will strike, and I will add fresh herbs, in this case thyme. Then I boil, watch, wait, and strain. Surprise—I have a syrup of epic proportions that is bracingly refreshing.

Juice the citrus into a saucepan; you should have about 1 cup of juice total. Add the water and thyme. Over medium heat, bring the liquid to a strong simmer. Cook for about 25 minutes, or until it is reduced by half. Do not stir.

Fill 2 glasses with ice or frozen berries, add $1/4$ cup of syrup to each and top off with seltzer water. Garnish with a slice of lemon or other citrus.

PER SERVING: Serving Size: 1 cup; Calories: 70; Total Fat: 0 g (0 g saturated, 0 g monounsaturated); Carbohydrates: 18 g; Protein: 1 g; Fiber: 3 g; Sodium: 1.5 mg

STORAGE: Store the syrup in an airtight container in the refrigerator for up to 1 week.

1 grapefruit

1 Meyer lemon

1 orange

1 cup filtered water

8 sprigs fresh thyme or lemon thyme

1 tablespoon honey or coconut palm sugar (optional)

Frozen berries (optional)

2 cups seltzer water

Lemon or other citrus slices, for garnish

Simon's Genius Elixir

MAKES 3 QUARTS • PREP TIME: 5 minutes • COOK TIME: 45 minutes

Let me tell you about Simon. Simon is thirteen. He's also a freaking genius when it comes to mixing healthy drinks. He comes by his knowledge of spices and fruits honestly; he's cooked in the kitchen with his dad, Jeremy, since he was a toddler. Even so, when Simon sent me this recipe, I was at first skeptical: boiled peaches, cardamom pods . . . I was, like, "where's 'eye of newt?'" Fear not; this drink is awesome and beautiful. It's like a quenching watercolor. That's because instead of grinding up the ingredients and creating a murky mess, you throw everything in whole. It looks like peach sangria and tastes heavenly, and the ginger has been shown to promote mental clarity. So, drinking the concoction of a genius can help make you a genius.

8 cups filtered water

1 cup peeled and sliced peaches

1 cinnamon stick, or
1 tablespoon ground
cinnamon

5 cardamom pods

4 allspice berries, or
$1/2$ teaspoon ground allspice

2 slices fresh ginger, or
1 teaspoon ground ginger

1 tablespoon organic coconut
palm sugar

1 tablespoon tart cherry juice,
or $1/4$ cup cherries

$1/4$ teaspoon vanilla extract

Pinch of salt

A few sprigs of mint

Put the water, peaches, cinnamon, cardamom, allspice, and ginger in a saucepan and bring to a boil over medium-high heat. Decrease the heat to low, cover, and simmer for 45 minutes.

Strain through a fine-mesh sieve. Stir in the coconut palm sugar, cherry juice, vanilla, and salt, stirring to dissolve the sugar, and cool completely.

Serve over ice with a sprig of mint and an extra teaspoon of cherry juice to create a sunset at the bottom of your glass.

VARIATION: Make this into a concentrated syrup by reducing the liquid over medium heat for an additional 20 minutes. You'll end up with about $1/3$ cup of syrup. Cool completely and serve over ice with seltzer or mineral water, or drizzle over yogurt.

PER SERVING: Serving Size: 1 cup; Calories: 36; Total Fat: 0 g (0 g saturated, 0 g monounsaturated); Carbohydrates: 9 g; Protein: 0.5 g; Fiber: 1 g; Sodium: 38 mg

STORAGE: Store in an airtight container in the refrigerator for up to 1 week.

Almond Milk

MAKES ABOUT 1 QUART • PREP TIME: 5 minutes • COOK TIME: Not applicable

The term *milk* has gone light-years beyond what it was when many of us were kids. No longer is the cow the only source, and that's a good thing—it gives us many more options. Whether because of taste preference, a desire to avoid dairy laced with excess hormones, lactose intolerance, or allergies, lots of folks are turning to alternative milks. One of my favorites is almond milk, because it's full of brain-boosting fats. The taste is also phenomenal, and it's phenomenally easy to make: a little soaking overnight, a run through the blender with some water, a quick strain through a nut bag (see Cook's Notes) and you've got a creamy milk that even Elsie would envy.

Soak the almonds in water to cover overnight.

Strain the almonds and rinse, then put them in a blender. Put the filtered water into a large measuring cup. Pour enough of the water into the blender to cover the almonds. Blend on high for 1 to 2 minutes, until the almonds are a smooth, creamy consistency. Hold a nut milk bag (see Cook's Note) over the measuring cup containing the remaining water, pour the blended almonds into the bag. Squeeze the bag gently at first to squeeze out most of the milk. Continue to firmly squeeze until no more liquid is extracted. Stir in a pinch of salt, then taste and add a bit more if necessary.

1 cup almonds

3 1/2 cups filtered water

Sea salt

VARIATIONS: If you'd like a little sweetness in your almond milk, add any of the following to the blender: half or one whole date, pitted, or 1/2 to 1 teaspoon of maple syrup or vanilla. If you want to take it over the top, add 1/2 teaspoon of cinnamon.

COOK'S NOTES: A nut milk bag is a special sack you can use to strain nut milks. The fine mesh keeps any sediment from getting into your milk.

Almond milk is a great alternative for use in Green Tea Chai (page 202), Brain-Berry Smoothie (page 207), or Mexican Hot Chocolate (page 200).

PER SERVING: Serving Size: 1 cup; Calories: 27.5; Total Fat: 1.5 g (0 g saturated, 0 g monounsaturated); Carbohydrates: 3.86 g; Protein: 0.5 g; Fiber: 0.5 g; Sodium: 73 mg

STORAGE: Store in an airtight container for up to 5 days.

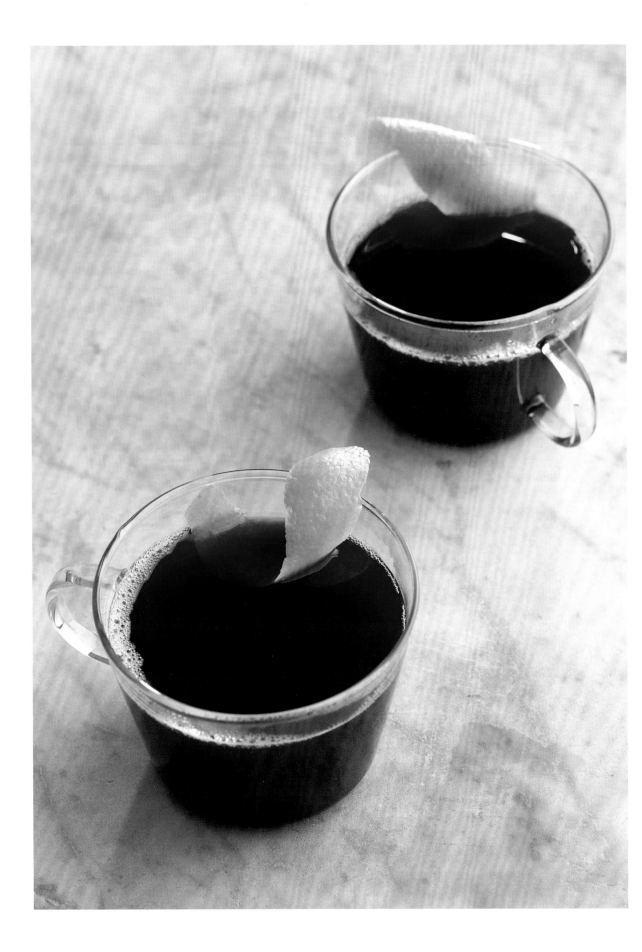

Jeanne's Brain Tea

MAKES ABOUT 1 QUART · PREP TIME: 5 · COOK TIME: 15 minutes

There's a lot of science going on in this tea, which is fitting because it was contributed by one of my favorite scientists, Jeanne Wallace, PhD. Jeanne knows everything about the brain, and she based this tea on the protective effects of certain berry extracts and green tea. It's so delicious that it works either hot or cold, and I especially like that the blueberry juice doesn't spike blood sugar, such spikes being a cause of fatigue and fuzziness. This brew of berries, orange peel, and cinnamon sticks comes together in just 15 minutes, and you'll often find a thermos of it cuddling up to me in the car on those long (honk-honk, beep-beep) California commutes.

Bring the water to a boil, add the tea bags, cinnamon, and orange peel. Turn off the heat and let steep for 3 minutes, then remove the tea bags, leaving the other ingredients to steep as the tea cools to room temperature. Remove the cinnamon stick and orange peel, strain into a glass pitcher, and add the berry concentrates. Drink warm or chilled. If desired, use sweetener.

COOK'S NOTES: Using a paring knife, peel the orange just above the bitter white pith.

Use some frozen blueberries as your ice cubes.

PER SERVING: Serving Size: 1 cup; Calories: 13; Total Fat: 0 g (0 g saturated, 0 g monounsaturated); Carbohydrates: 3 g; Protein: 0 g; Fiber: 1 g; Sodium: 6 mg

STORAGE: Store in an airtight container in the refrigerator for up to 1 week.

4 cups filtered water

4 organic green tea bags

1 cinnamon stick

Peel of 1 small organic orange, or 2 teaspoons dried organic citrus peel

3 tablespoons unsweetened blueberry juice concentrate

3 tablespoons unsweetened concentrate of another juice such as raspberry, tart cherry, black currant, cranberry, lingonberry, or pomegranate

Sweetener (optional)

Hazelnut Milk

MAKES 1 QUART · PREP TIME: 5 minutes (after overnight soaking) · COOK TIME: Not applicable

Hazelnuts get a bad rap in America, and I can understand why. They're often found in cheap, packaged nut mixes that are years old and, consequently, rancid. This is a shame, because a fresh hazelnut is a delight to behold. The rest of the world knows this, as hazelnuts enjoy tremendous popularity in places such as Turkey, Italy, and France. They're the toasty kick in pralines, the heady ambiance in Frangelico, the yin to chocolate's yang in Nutella, and they give this milk a bevy of fats, minerals, and vitamins that benefit the brain (notably vitamin E, which may help prevent cognitive decline). With a nine-thousand-year history, hazelnuts are no Johnny-come-lately, but they sure may keep Johnny smart.

1 cup hazelnuts

3$\frac{1}{2}$ cups filtered water

Sea salt

Soak the hazelnuts in water overnight.

Strain the hazelnuts and rinse, then put them in the blender. Put the filtered water in a large measuring cup. Pour enough of the water into the blender to cover the almonds. Blend on high for 1 to 2 minutes, until the hazelnuts are a smooth, creamy consistency. Hold a nut milk bag (see Cook's Notes, page 195) over the measuring cup with the remaining water and pour the blended hazelnuts into the bag. Squeeze the bag gently at first to squeeze out most of the milk. Continue to firmly squeeze until no more liquid is extracted. Stir in a pinch of salt, then taste and add a bit more if necessary.

VARIATIONS: If you'd like a little sweetness in your hazelnut milk, add any of the following to the blender: half to one whole date, pitted, or $\frac{1}{2}$ to 1 teaspoon of maple syrup or vanilla.

To go above and beyond, add 1 teaspoon of unsweetened cocoa powder or a grating of nutmeg.

PER SERVING: Serving Size: 1 cup; Calories: 62; Total Fat: 3 g (1 g saturated, 2 g monounsaturated); Carbohydrates: 7 g; Protein: 1 g; Fiber: 0 g; Sodium: 30 mg

STORAGE: Store in an airtight container in the refrigerator for up to 5 days.

Cafe Mocha
WITH HAZELNUT MILK

MAKES 1 SERVING • PREP TIME: 5 minutes • COOK TIME: 5 minutes

---

Someone asked me why we were doing coffees in this book. Truth is, coffee drinkers love their joe, and a little bit of caffeine is good—and energizing—for the brain's dopamine receptors. That said, the motto in the Katz kitchen is, if you're going to do something, do it right. Instead of store-bought mochas—which, if you add syrup, contain who-knows-how-much sugar or corn syrup—our way is to combine top-notch cocoa powder, a hit of coffee or espresso, a half-cup of steamed hazelnut milk (page 198) for that special heady taste, and a pinch of cinnamon or a cinnamon stick. I swear this is like drinking a candy bar minus the sugar. Trust me. Try it.

Put the cocoa powder in the bottom of a coffee cup. Add the coffee and top with the hazelnut milk and dash of cinnamon.

VARIATION: Jeanne's Pumpkin Pie Spiced Latte: combine $3/4$ cup of frothed coconut milk, 2 tablespoons of maple syrup, $1/4$ teaspoon of pumpkin spice, and a double shot of espresso.

COOK'S NOTE: Both almond milk and hazelnut milk will separate slightly because of the acidity of the coffee. Foaming the froth will hide that and add mouthfeel, so you can enjoy your dairy-free latte.

$1/2$ teaspoon unsweetened cocoa powder

$3/4$ cup brewed coffee or 1 to 2 shots espresso

$1/2$ cup Hazelnut Milk (page 198) or store-bought organic hazelnut milk, steamed or warmed

Dash of cinnamon and/or nutmeg

PER SERVING: Serving Size: 1 cup; Calories: 61; Total Fat: 2 g (0 g saturated, 0 g monounsaturated); Carbohydrates: 10 g; Protein: 1.5 g; Fiber: 1 g; Sodium: 64 mg

STORAGE: Not applicable

Mexican Hot Chocolate

MAKES 1 SERVING · PREP TIME: 5 minutes · COOK TIME: Not applicable

How do you improve on something that's practically perfect? Take it south of the border! This isn't the hot chocolate of the days of yore (not that we complained back then), when you used to write your name in the milk with the syrup; this is far healthier and, hard as it may be to believe, far tastier. This is like eating an almond chocolate bar with a zing, as almond milk combines with cocoa, cinnamon, and cayenne to add some culinary heat to this most favorite of hot drinks.

1 cup Almond Milk (page 195) or store-bought unsweetened almond milk

1 tablespoon unsweetened cocoa powder

2 teaspoons Grade B maple syrup

1/4 teaspoon ground cinnamon

Pinch of sea salt

Pinch of cayenne

In a sauce pan over low heat, warm the almond milk. Whisk in the cocoa powder, maple syrup, cinnamon, salt, and cayenne and simmer, whisking constantly, for about 1 minute or until slightly thickened. The liquid should coat the back of a spoon. Pour into a cup and serve.

VARIATIONS: If you want a hot Nutella drink, use Hazelnut Milk (page 198) instead of almond milk and add a grating of nutmeg in addition to the other spices. You also might like this with coconut milk.

COOK'S NOTE: The key to this drink is using a whisk. Whisking aerates the milk, transforming it into a luscious creamy cup of yum!

PER SERVING: Serving Size: 1 cup; Calories: 42; Total Fat: 2 g (0 g saturated, 0 g monounsaturated); Carbohydrates: 6 g; Protein: 1 g; Fiber: 1 g; Sodium: 173 mg

STORAGE: Not applicable

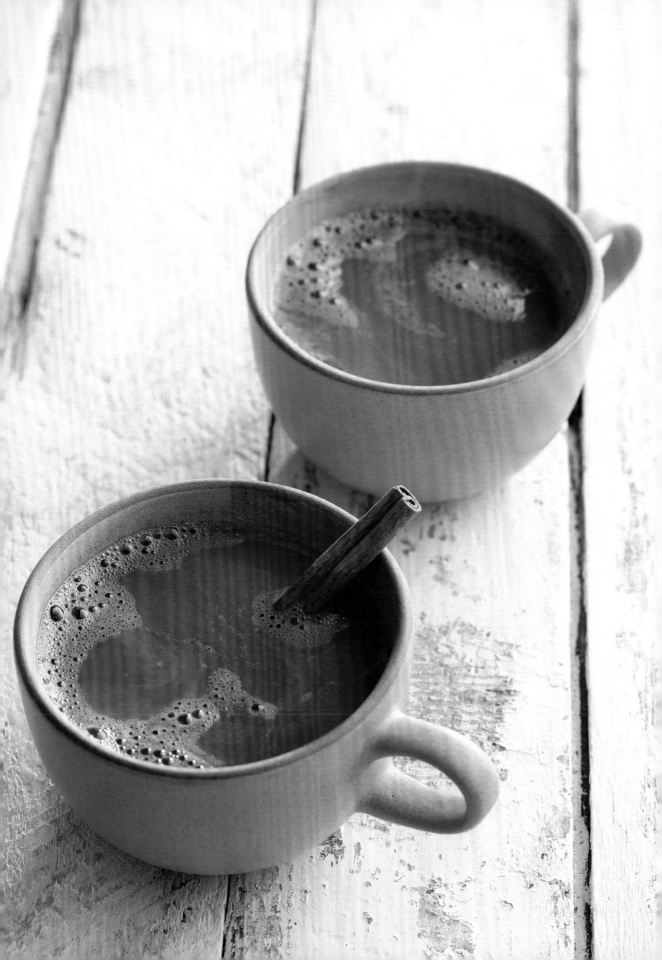

Green Tea Chai

MAKES 3 QUARTS · PREP TIME: 5 minutes · COOK TIME: 45 minutes

How do I love thee? By keeping thee at all times on my refrigerator shelf. Seriously. My husband, Gregg, lives on iced tea, and he loves this green chai in particular. Green tea is a real brain-boosting food, and here we up the ante by adding ginger, cinnamon, and coriander, all of which have top-notch anti-inflammatory properties. In our house, this is a go-to for staying sharp throughout the day.

3 quarts filtered water

1/3 cup sliced peeled fresh ginger

3 tablespoons coriander seeds

1 1/2 tablespoons cardamom pods

4 cinnamon sticks

5 whole cloves

4 green tea bags

In a saucepan, combine 2 quarts of the water with the ginger, coriander, cardamom, cinnamon, and cloves and bring to a boil over high heat. Lower the heat to medium low, cover, and simmer for 45 minutes.

While the chai spice mixture is simmering, make the green tea. In a large saucepan, bring the remaining 4 cups of water to a boil over high heat, then add the tea bags. Steep for 6 minutes.

Remove the tea bags and discard them and strain the chai mixture through a fine-mesh sieve into the green tea. (Reserve the strained out spices; see the Cook's Note.)

VARIATION: To make a green tea chai latte, combine 1/2 cup of green chai tea with 1/2 cup of Almond Milk (page 195) or Hazelnut Milk (page 198) and 1 to 3 tablespoons of maple syrup and gently heat for 2 to 3 minutes (don't boil). Stir in 1 teaspoon of vanilla, then taste. Add more milk or sweetener if you like, and serve hot or cold.

COOK'S NOTE: Keep the spices that are strained out of the tea and use them to make another, smaller batch of tea. The spices will keep in the refrigerator for 4 to 5 days and in the freezer for a month. To make more tea, combine the spices and 6 cups of water and bring to a boil. Add 2 tablespoons of peeled fresh ginger slices. Simmer for 30 minutes, then strain the tea and discard the spices.

PER SERVING: Serving Size: 1 cup; Calories: 11; Total Fat: 0.5 g (0 g saturated, 0 g monounsaturated); Carbohydrates: 2 g; Protein: 0 g; Fiber: 0 g; Sodium: 16 mg

STORAGE: Store in an airtight container in the refrigerator for 2 weeks.

Mellow Kudzu Elixir

MAKES 1 SERVING · PREP TIME: 3 minutes · COOK TIME: 5 minutes

If this were the 1960s, I'd call this the "ohmmmmm" elixir, as kudzu root has a way of eliciting a meditative state. Now, we'd just call it "chill," because that's certainly what kudzu does in this drink, thickening spiced apple juice slightly to a silky consistency. This is a variation of the tried and true recipe by my mentor, Annemarie Colbin, who was looking for ways to make puddings that didn't require milk or eggs, and turned to kudzu. It thickens the same way as cornstarch does—by being dissolved in a cold liquid and then heated while you stir it. After a few days of eating it for breakfast, she began to realize she was feeling exceedingly mellow and sleeping really well. And you didn't hear this from me, but this elixir makes for a heckuva hangover remedy.

In a small pot, mix the kudzu into the cold apple juice, stirring until dissolved. Stir in the ginger, vanilla, and cinnamon, then turn the burner on and bring to a gentle boil over medium heat, stirring constantly, until the liquid thickens and becomes translucent, about 5 minutes. Serve hot or cold.

VARIATIONS: For a cozy and soothing pudding that's closer to Annemarie's original recipe, leave out the ginger and cinnamon and increase the amount of kudzu to 2 tablespoons.

For a more nutrient-dense pudding, swirl 1 tablespoon of tahini into the mixture as soon as it thickens.

PER SERVING: Serving Size: 1 cup; Calories: 181; Total Fat: 0 g (0 g saturated, 0 g monounsaturated); Carbohydrates: 43 g; Protein: 0 g; Fiber: 0.5 g; Sodium: 6 mg

STORAGE: Not applicable

$1^{1}/_{2}$ tablespoons kudzu root powder

1 cup cold unfiltered apple juice

$^{1}/_{8}$ teaspoon grated fresh ginger (optional)

1 teaspoon vanilla extract

$^{1}/_{4}$ teaspoon ground cinnamon

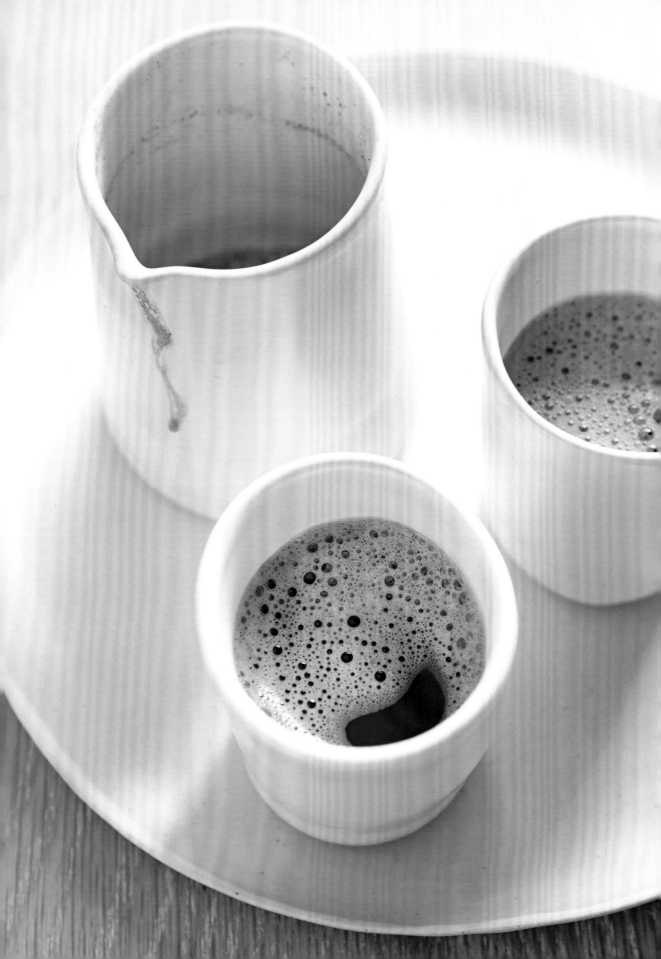

Eric Gower's Perfect Cup of Matcha

MAKES 1 SERVING · PREP TIME: 5 minutes · COOK TIME: 5 minutes

If you're not familiar with *matcha*, it's a finely powdered green tea. And if you're not familiar with chef Eric Gower, his *matcha* is to green tea as Dom Perignon is to Champagne. Eric spent sixteen years in Japan learning the customs and history behind one of the healthiest teas on the planet. I took a class with him and he made me a *matcha* convert; now, every day at 3 p.m. on days when we're home working, my husband, Gregg, and I stop everything for a few minutes and do a little tea ceremony around this hearty brew. I thank you, Eric, for allowing me to share your *matcha* method with my readers. We all give you a virtual bow.

The perfect cup of *matcha* is like making the perfect cup of expresso, so you will need some special equipment here, including a small fine-mesh sieve or sifter, a *matcha* scoop (use a teaspoon if you don't have one), a frother (see Cook's Notes, next page), and a mug.

Place a small fine-mesh sieve or strainer over a deep mug. Scoop the *matcha* into the sieve and gently shake it allow the *matcha* to fall through. Then gently push the remainder through the sieve with your *matcha* scoop or a teaspoon.

1/4 cup boiled filtered water
1/2 to 1 teaspoon matcha

Fill a small teacup with 1/4 cup of the boiled water and let it sit for one minute. Transfer the hot water from the small cup to the mug with the sifted *matcha* in it. Swirl it around like wine, and, using the tip of the frother, scrape around the bottom to make sure no clumps remain.

Tilt the mug at a pretty steep angle and turn on the frother. Insert the frother deep down to mix everything thoroughly for just a few seconds, trying not to hit the side of the mug—just froth the liquid. Then bring the tip of the frother up a bit, so that you're frothing the froth, not so much the water. The whole act of frothing should take no longer than 8 to 10 seconds (additional frothing doesn't create better *crema*). Swirl the *matcha*, as you would a glass of wine, and give it a few firm taps to pop any large bubbles. Then pour it back into the smaller, preheated cup, and serve.

CONTINUED

Eric Gower's Perfect Cup of Matcha, *continued*

COOK'S NOTES: Filling the small cup with boiling water and transferring it to the larger mug accomplishes three important things: it preheats the cup, which will keep the *matcha* hotter for longer; it cools the boiled water to the desired brewing temperature of 175° to 180°F; and it premeasures your water.

According to Eric Gower, a nice cup of *matcha* would ideally have roughly two ounces (that is, a quarter-cup) of creamy, perfectly frothed green ambrosia, made in a small pitcher or creamer (or even a mug, as here), and then transferred to a small, elegant cup for serving. Achieving the *crema* means you using the right tool—a battery-operated handheld milk-foaming wand. With a little practice, you'll become a *matcha* barista, whipping up a cup of *matcha* with a dreamy *crema* every time.

PER SERVING: Calories: 5; Total Fat: 0 g (0 g saturated, 0 g monounsaturated); Carbohydrates: 0 g; Protein: 0.2 g; Fiber: 0.2 g; Sodium: 5 mg
STORAGE: Not applicable

Brain-Berry Smoothie

MAKES 1 QUART · PREP TIME: 5 minutes · COOK TIME: Not applicable

Here's a technical term for you: bioavailability. In this case, it means your body's ability to absorb the nutrients from various foods. Certain ingredients can make the nutrients in a dish more (or less) bioavailable: that's why all smoothies are not alike. If this smoothie were just ice, water, and berries, it would fly right through your system with nary a nutrient remaining behind. But with both good fats (almond butter and yogurt) and a little fiber (flaxseed) in the mix, all the phenomenal brain-protective anthocyanins in the blueberries, blackberries, and cherries are slowly absorbed into the body—and your blood sugar doesn't spike. Oh, and did I mention the taste? Superb! Take it along in a thermos to keep you rolling and productive throughout the day.

Combine the yogurt, water, lemon juice, and ginger in a blender and process until smooth. Add the blueberries, blackberries, cherries, almond butter, ground flaxseed, syrup, and salt and blend until smooth and creamy.

VARIATION: For more protein, add a scoop of whey protein powder.

COOK'S NOTE: Once the smoothie is well blended, keep blending this a little longer to be sure the blackberry seeds are all pulverized.

PER SERVING: Serving Size: 1 cup; Calories: 147; Total Fat: 8 g (2.5 g saturated, 2 g monounsaturated); Carbohydrates: 16 g; Protein: 6.5 g; Fiber: 6 g; Sodium: 22 mg

STORAGE: Not applicable

1 cup plain organic full-fat yogurt

1 cup filtered water

1 teaspoon freshly squeezed lemon juice

1 teaspoon grated ginger

1 cup fresh or frozen blueberries

1 cup fresh or frozen blackberries

1 cup fresh or frozen cherries, pitted and halved

3 tablespoons almond butter

1 tablespoon finely ground flaxseed

$1^1/_2$ teaspoons Grade B maple syrup

Pinch of sea salt

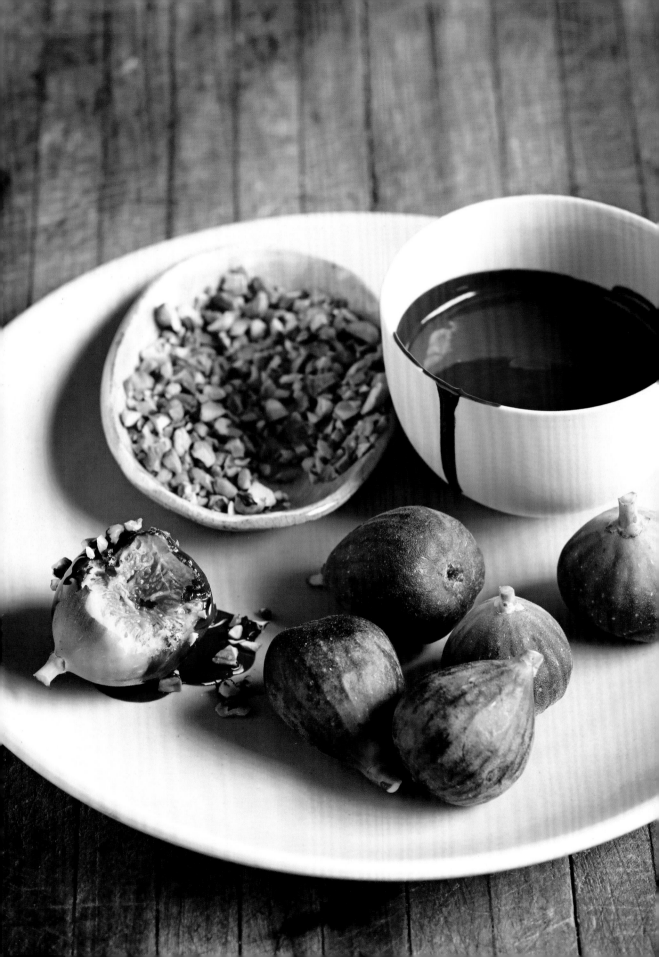

CHAPTER 10

Sweet Bites

As a psychologist friend of mine says, "Man cannot live on kale alone." We're hardwired to enjoy sugar; the key, of course, is choosing the right kinds of unrefined sugar and practicing moderation (that's my way of saying you can't go out and eat a jar of jelly beans just because your brain needs energy). There's no refined sugar in any of these sweet bites, nor is there any gluten. That's important for people with gluten sensitivities, as gluten consumption for them may cause a host of ailments, including depression, nerve damage, anxiety, and headaches. But what we did put in is amazing, in terms of both taste and satiation, balancing good fats and fiber to go along with the sweet, meaning you'll feel full after just a few bites and avoid the brain fog that comes with a sugar overload. I'm proud of the creativity of my talented colleagues who helped me come up with inventing these goodies: there's something here for everyone, and the ingredients offer a host of antioxidant and anti-inflammatory brain benefits. (Did I mention that chocolate is a mood elevator? Did I have to?!)

Slow-Roasted Spiced Peaches

MAKES ABOUT 1 CUP • PREP TIME: 10 minutes • COOK TIME: 1¹/₂ hours

I owe this one to my mom, who taught me all about peaches, in her own inimitable style. Didn't matter what peach dish she was making—peach kuchen, peach cake, peach you-name-it—Mom had a scrumptious way with peaches. These peaches are simple and absolutely intoxicating; take peaches at the height of their season and toss them with cinnamon, ginger, and just a spritz of lemon juice. You'll find yourself making excuses to be in the kitchen while these goodies roast, cause they just smell *soooooo* good. Thanks, Mom! These can be served with the Blackberry Parfaits with Sesame Brittle (page 217). Triple this recipe and use it to fill a cashew crust (see page 213), or keep it simple and spoon them over Greek yogurt.

1 tablespoon Grade B maple syrup

1¹/₂ teaspoons extra-virgin olive oil

1 teaspoon freshly squeezed lemon juice

¹/₄ teaspoon sea salt

¹/₄ teaspoon ground cinnamon

1 teaspoon freshly grated ginger, or 1¹/₂ teaspoons ground

4 peaches, peeled and sliced

2 teaspoons very thinly sliced fresh mint

Preheat the oven to 300°F. Line a rimmed baking sheet with parchment paper.

Put the maple syrup, olive oil, lemon juice, salt, cinnamon, and ginger in a large bowl and whisk to combine. Add the peaches and stir gently until they are well coated.

Spread the peaches on the lined baking sheet in a single layer. Bake for about 1¹/₂ hours, until the peaches are moist and about a third their original size, stirring and redistributing them halfway through the baking time. Let cool for 5 minutes, then transfer the peaches and any remaining juices to a bowl. Gently stir in the mint, then let sit for 5 minutes for the flavors to meld. Serve warm or at room temperature.

PER SERVING: Serving Size: ¹/₂ cup; Calories: 189; Total Fat: 4 g (1 g saturated, 3 g monounsaturated); Carbohydrates: 20 g; Protein: 2 g; Fiber: 3 g; Sodium: 204 mg

STORAGE: Store in an airtight container in the refrigerator for up to 2 days or in the freezer for up to 3 months.

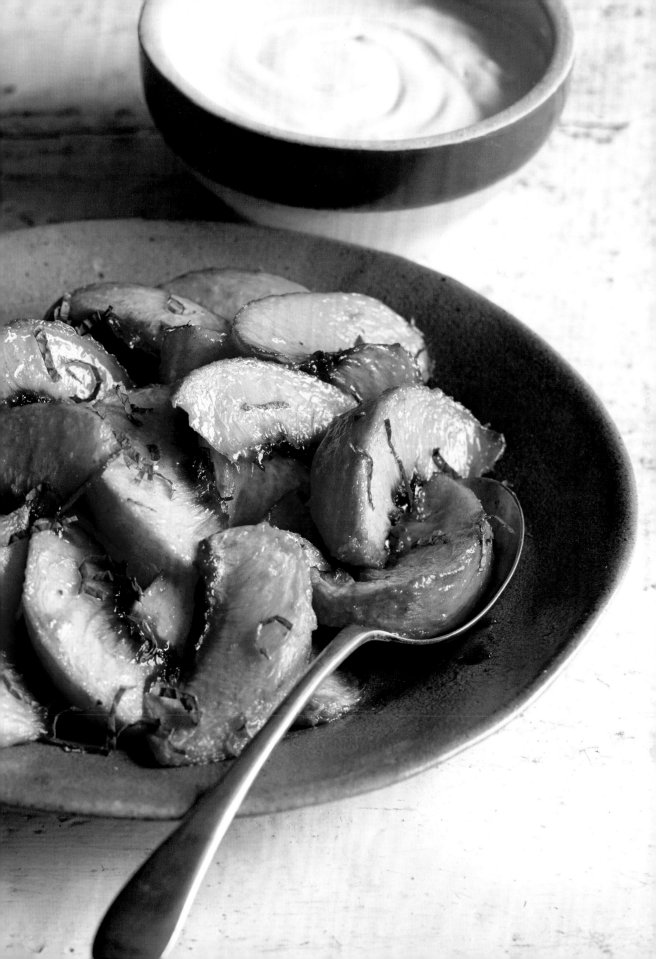

Campfire Style Seasonal Fruit Fondue
WITH CHOCOLATE

MAKES 4 SERVINGS • PREP TIME: 10 minutes • COOK TIME: 5 minutes

At our house we firmly believe that chocolate—brain-boosting, mood-enhancing chocolate—goes with anything. Doesn't matter what time of year: take a seasonal fruit and nut combo for a chocolate dip and it invariably shows taste bud superpowers. Starting in the fall, we pair pears and almonds, then move into winter with a banana-walnut duet. Spring blooms with strawberries and macadamia nuts, while summer serves up cherries and almonds. And just because I can, I'm delivering on an unofficial fifth season—call it Indian summer—where figs and pistachios take to the plate, thus proving that no matter what hemisphere you inhabit, chocolate never goes out of season.

FALL

2 ripe but firm pears, halved, cored, each half sliced into 6 slices

2 tablespoons finely chopped toasted almonds

WINTER

2 bananas, peeled and sliced diagonally

2 tablespoons finely chopped toasted walnuts

SPRING

1 pint strawberries

2 tablespoons finely chopped toasted macadamias

SUMMER

2 cups cherries with stems

2 tablespoons finely chopped toasted almonds

LATE SUMMER

12 fresh figs

2 tablespoons finely chopped toasted pistachios

3 ounces dark chocolate (at least 68% cacao content), finely chopped

1/2 teaspoon grapeseed oil

Tiny pinch of salt

Arrange the fruit on a serving plate and place the nuts in a small bowl. Place the chopped chocolate in a pan or bowl set over another pan with a little boiling water. Add the oil and salt and stir until melted and smooth. Transfer the chocolate mixture into a bowl and serve alongside the fruit and nuts. To eat, dunk a piece of fruit into the chocolate and sprinkle with nuts.

COOK'S NOTE: To create individual dessert plates, dip separate pieces of fruit in the melted chocolate. Place them on a parchment-lined sheet pan and sprinkle with a pinch or two of nuts. Allow to cool slightly before serving.

PER SERVING: Calories: 88; Total Fat: 5g (2 g saturated, 3 g monounsaturated); Carbohydrates: 15 g; Protein: 1 g; Fiber: 3 g; Sodium: 6 mg

STORAGE: Not applicable

Pumpkin Tart in a Cashew Crust

MAKES 12 SERVINGS • PREP TIME: 20 minutes • COOK TIME: 1 hour 15 minutes

This one was a culinary conundrum: how to make a certifiably delicious, completely over-the-top pumpkin filling *without* the refined sugar blast of condensed milk in pumpkin pie filling? The answer was in a combination of molasses and coconut milk, which gives the kind of mouthfeel that had my husband, Gregg (who considers pumpkin its own food group), giving this recipe a thumbs-up. If you haven't encountered the gluten-free grain teff before, it's a true nutritional powerhouse—and the tiniest whole grain in the world; a hundred grains of teff equal one wheat kernel. I love teff's light, nutty taste, which perfectly complements the cashews in this tart.

Preheat the oven to 375°F. Lightly grease 9-inch pie plate with a neutral oil.

To make the crust, in the bowl of a food processor, combine the cashews, teff flour, baking powder, and salt. Process until the cashews are broken into fine bits. Transfer the mixture to a bowl and add the ghee and maple syrup; stir to combine well. Spoon the mixture into the prepared pan and, using your fingers, press firmly into a thin and even layer to the top of the pan. Bake for 15 minutes. It will have puffed up a bit, so cool on a cooling rack for 10 minutes before filling. It will settle into the pan.

Increase the oven temperature to 400°F. To make the filling, in a large bowl or stand mixer, lightly beat the eggs (they should not get foamy). Add pumpkin, salt, cinnamon, ginger, cloves, allspice, and nutmeg and stir to combine. Mix in the maple syrup, molasses, and coconut milk. Pour into the warm tart shell and bake for 15 minutes.

Reduce the oven temperature to 350°F and continue baking for another 30 to 40 minutes, until the filling no longer jiggles and has small cracks in the surface.

Serve in thin slices.

COOK'S NOTE: If the crust puffs up on the initial baking and doesn't flatten while it's cooling, use the back of a fork to press it down.

PER SERVING: Serving Size: 1 slice; Calories: 311; Total Fat: 22 g (11 g saturated, 6 g monounsaturated); Carbohydrates: 25 g; Protein: 7 g; Fiber: 3 g; Sodium: 183 mg

STORAGE: Store covered in the refrigerator for up to 5 days or in the freezer for up to 1 month.

CRUST

1 1/2 cups cashews

3/4 cup teff flour (see Resources)

1/2 teaspoon baking powder

1/2 teaspoon salt

1/4 cup ghee, melted

3 tablespoons Grade B maple syrup

FILLING

2 organic eggs

1 (15-ounce) can organic pumpkin

1/2 teaspoon sea salt

1 teaspoon cinnamon

1/2 teaspoon ground ginger

1/4 teaspoon ground cloves

1/4 teaspoon ground allspice

1/4 teaspoon freshly grated nutmeg

3 tablespoons Grade B maple syrup

3 tablespoons molasses

1 (13.66-ounce) can full-fat coconut milk

Chocolate Cherry Walnut Truffles

MAKES ABOUT 20 TRUFFLES • PREP TIME: 15 minutes • COOK TIME: 2¼ hours

My dad, Jay, had this delightful habit; whenever you told him something that struck his fancy, he'd roar, "That's FANTASTIC!" and gleefully clap his hands for emphasis. This was doubly true if you told him he was getting chocolate for dessert. Jay never met a piece of chocolate he didn't like, and I have a feeling that just hearing what's in these truffles—dates, cherries, and walnuts, smothered in chocolate, rolled in coconut and curry—would've given him cause to offer up a standing ovation. Studies suggest walnuts may boost memory, while chocolate, as we all know, is the ultimate mood-boosting agent. One bite of this dessert and you'd be hard-pressed to feel any stress.

2 tablespoons boiling water

2 ounces dark chocolate (64 to 72% cacao content), very finely chopped

½ cup walnuts

1 tablespoon unsweetened cocoa powder

1 cup pitted and halved Medjool dates

1 teaspoon vanilla extract

Sea salt

¼ cup finely diced dried cherries

2 tablespoons shredded coconut

¼ teaspoon curry powder

Stir the boiling water into the chopped chocolate and let it stand for 30 seconds. Using a small whisk, stir until the chocolate is completely melted and glossy.

Coarsely grind the walnuts in a food processor, then add the cocoa powder, dates, vanilla, and ⅛ teaspoon of salt, and process for a minute. Then add the chocolate mixture and process until smooth, another minute. Transfer to a bowl and stir the cherries into the chocolate mixture. Cover and chill for approximately 2 hours, until firm.

On a plate, mix the coconut, curry powder, and a pinch of salt. Scoop up approximately 2 teaspoons of the chilled chocolate mixture and roll it into a smooth ball between your palms, then roll it in the curried coconuts to coat. Repeat with the remaining mixture, then place the truffles in an airtight container and chill thoroughly before serving.

COOK'S NOTE: If you want to give the truffles a golden hue, toast the coconut in a 300°F oven for 10 to 15 minutes.

PER SERVING: Serving Size: 1 truffle; Calories: 72; Total Fat: 4 g (1 g saturated, 1 g monounsaturated); Carbohydrates: 9 g; Protein: 1 g; Fiber: 1 g; Sodium: 16 mg

STORAGE: Store in an airtight container for 2 days

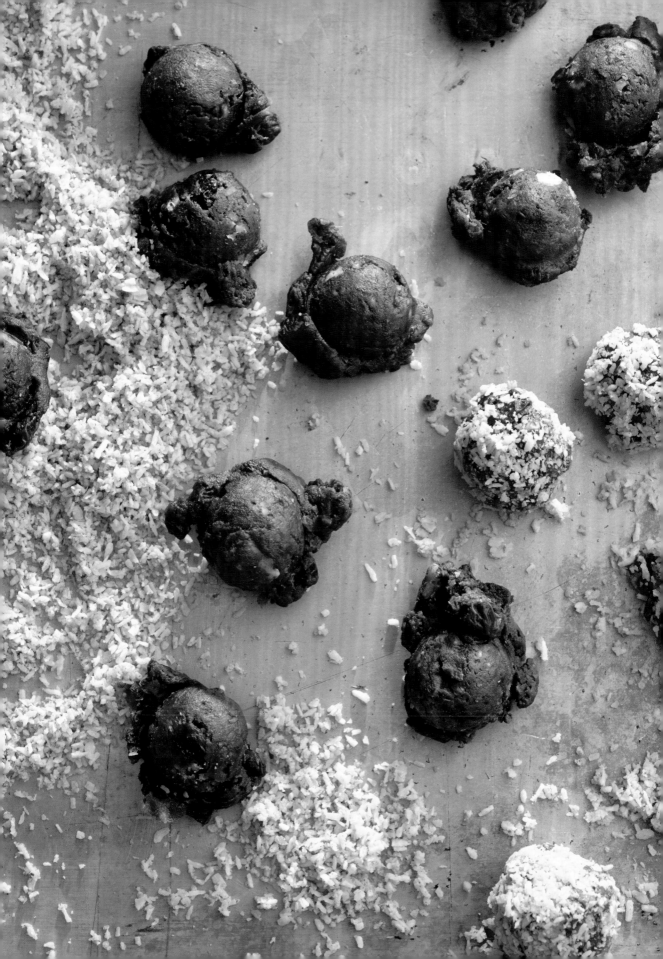

Fall Pear Crisp

MAKES 6 SERVINGS • PREP TIME: 20 minutes • COOK TIME: 1 hour

Every season needs a crisp; this is my homage to fall. I use two different pears, Anjou and Bosc, for their slightly different consistency and taste. Cranberries add just the right amount of sweet and tart. An added bonus: cranberries benefit the brain's synapses.

FILLING

4 Anjou pears, peeled, cored, and cubed

2 Bosc pears, peeled, cored, and cubed

1/4 cup dried cranberries

1 tablespoon minced fresh ginger

2 tablespoons freshly squeezed lemon juice

2 tablespoons water

1 tablespoon Grade B maple syrup

3/4 teaspoon ground cinnamon

1/4 teaspoon sea salt

TOPPING

1 cup coarsely chopped walnuts

3/4 cup coarsely chopped pecans

1/2 cup sunflower seeds

1/2 cup pumpkin seeds

1/3 cup coconut oil or ghee, melted

1/4 cup unsweetened shredded coconut or coconut flour

1/2 cup gluten-free rolled oats

3 tablespoons Grade B maple syrup

1/2 teaspoon ground cinnamon

1/2 teaspoon sea salt

Preheat the oven to 400°F.

To make the filling, combine the pears, cranberries, ginger, lemon juice, water, syrup, cinnamon, and salt in a large bowl and toss until the fruit is well coated. Transfer the fruit mixture to a 2-quart baking dish or a 10-inch pie plate.

To make the topping, combine the walnuts, pecans, sunflower seeds, pumpkin seeds, oil, coconut, oats, syrup, cinnamon, and salt in a large bowl and stir until well combined. Spoon the topping evenly over the filling and lightly press with your fingers until the fruit is covered and the dish is full. Cover the dish with foil and bake for about 40 minutes, until the fruit is soft. Remove the foil and continue to bake for another 15 to 20 minutes, until the topping is golden and the filling is bubbly. Let cool for at least 10 minutes. Serve warm or at room temperature.

PER SERVING: Serving Size: 1 cup; Calories: 361; Total Fat: 25 g (8 g saturated, 4 g monounsaturated); Carbohydrates: 31.5 g; Protein: 7 g; Fiber: 7 g; Sodium: 137 mg

STORAGE: Store in an airtight container in the refrigerator for up to 4 days.

Blackberry Parfaits
WITH SESAME BRITTLE

MAKES 4 SERVINGS · PREP TIME: 10 minutes · COOK TIME: 20 minutes

This is layered yum in a cup. The blackberries are a compote, which become sweeter by the minute as it boils down to a warm sauce. It alternates in the cup with layers of luscious Greek yogurt, which is full of probiotics. The sesame-maple brittle is the final touch, adding a bit of crunch. So pretty.

To make the compote, combine the blackberries, orange juice, zest, syrup, and ginger in a small saucepan over medium heat. Cook, stirring occasionally, for 3 to 4 minutes, until the mixture bubbles, pulls away from the sides of the pan, and becomes syrupy. Remove from the heat and set aside.

To make the brittle, preheat the oven to 375°F and turn the oven light on. Line a rimmed baking sheet with parchment paper. Spread the oil on the parchment paper with a paper towel, covering the parchment with a thin, even film of oil.

Put the maple syrup, sesame seeds, cardamom, and salt in a small bowl. Pour the mixture onto the oiled parchment paper, then tilt the pan to spread it evenly. Bake for 5 to 7 minutes, staying close to the oven and keeping watch. The syrup will first become bubbly, then, after another 2 or 3 minutes, the sesame seeds will take on a nice golden color and the syrup will turn a deep amber color. At this point, remove the brittle from the oven and let it cool to room temperature.

Using a thin metal spatula, lift the hardened brittle and break it into randomly sized pieces. (To make it easier to break into pieces, you can pop it into the freezer for about 5 minutes.) Use immediately or store in an airtight container.

Fill each of 4 parfait glasses with 1 tablespoon of compote, then $1/4$ cup of yogurt, then 1 tablespoon of compote, then $1/4$ cup of yogurt, and top with a piece of the sesame brittle.

VARIATIONS: If you have fresh blackberries, all the better. Just add 2 tablespoons of water to the recipe. If you don't have blackberries, use blueberries, strawberries, and/or raspberries.

PER SERVING: Serving Size: $1/2$ cup yogurt, 2 tablespoons compote; Calories: 143; Total Fat: 1 g (0 g saturated, 0 g monounsaturated); Carbohydrates: 39 g; Protein: 2 g; Fiber: 11 g; Sodium: 1 mg

STORAGE: Store in an airtight container in the refrigerator for 7 days or in the freezer for 2 months.

COMPOTE

$1^1/2$ cups frozen blackberries

1 teaspoon freshly squeezed orange or lemon juice

1 teaspoon orange or lemon zest

$1^1/2$ teaspoons Grade B maple syrup

$1/4$ teaspoon ground ginger

SESAME BRITTLE

1 scant teaspoon extra-virgin olive oil

3 tablespoons Grade B maple syrup

2 tablespoons sesame seeds

$1/8$ teaspoon ground cardamon

Pinch of sea salt

2 cups organic plain Greek yogurt

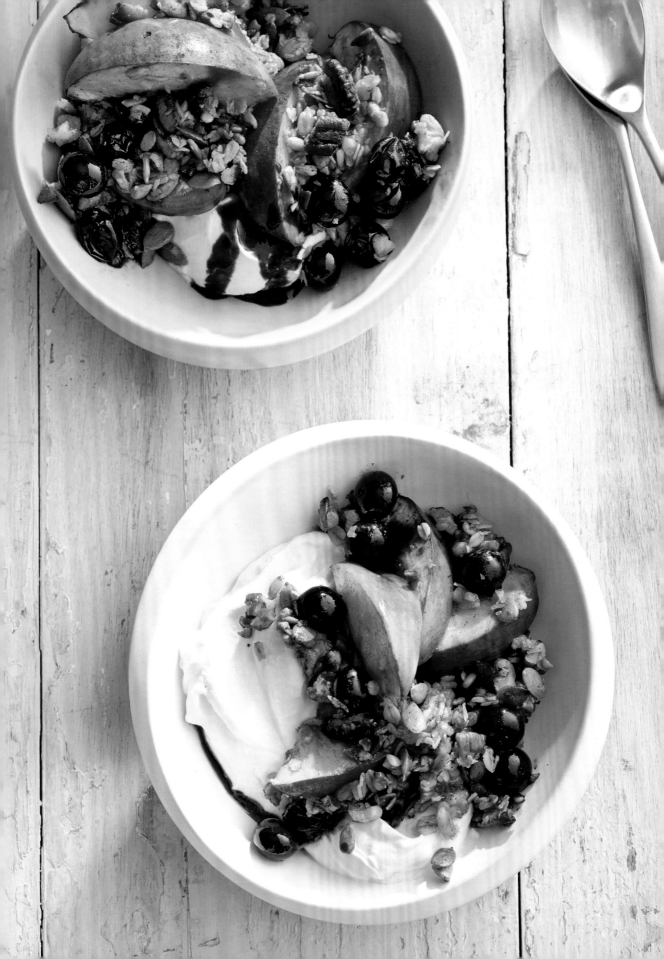

Julie's Best Nectarine Blueberry Crisp

MAKES 6 SERVINGS • PREP TIME: 20 minutes • COOK TIME: 40 minutes

Eating a crisp is heaven's way of saying you must have done something right (or nice) today. My cooking buddy, a serious baker, says crisps need to look "abundant." All I know is that her nectarine and blueberry crisps, which served as my inspiration here, take *abundant* to the limit. The smells that suffuse the kitchen as this dish bakes are absolutely intoxicating, nectarines and blueberries blending with coconut oil, cinnamon, and nuts to create an olfactory orgasm. (Can I say that? Wait, I just did!)

Preheat the oven to 375°F.

To make the filling, combine the nectarines, blueberries, salt, and cinnamon in a large bowl and toss until the fruit is well coated. Transfer the fruit mixture to a 2-quart baking dish or a 10-inch pie plate.

To make the topping, combine the walnuts, pecans, sunflower seeds, pumpkin seeds, oil, coconut, oats, syrup, cinnamon, and salt in a large bowl and stir well. Spoon the topping evenly over the filling and lightly press with your fingers until the fruit is covered and the dish is full. Bake for about 40 minutes, until the topping is golden and the filling is bubbly. Let cool for at least 10 minutes. Serve warm or at room temperature.

PER SERVING: Serving Size: 1 cup; Calories: 328; Total Fat: 25 g (8 g saturated, 4 g monounsaturated); Carbohydrates: 22 g; Protein: 7 g; Fiber: 5 g; Sodium: 136 mg

STORAGE: Store in an airtight container in the refrigerator for up to 3 days.

FILLING

8 nectarines, unpeeled and sliced into $1/2$-inch-thick wedges

3 cups blueberries

$1/4$ teaspoon sea salt

Pinch of ground cinnamon

TOPPING

1 cup coarsely chopped walnuts

$3/4$ cup coarsely chopped pecans

$1/2$ cup sunflower seeds

$1/2$ cup pumpkin seeds

$1/3$ cup coconut oil or ghee, melted

$1/4$ cup unsweetened shredded coconut or coconut flour

$1/2$ cup gluten-free rolled oats

3 tablespoons Grade B maple syrup

$1/2$ teaspoon ground cinnamon

$1/2$ teaspoon sea salt

Meyer Lemon Pudding
WITH FRESH STRAWBERRIES

MAKES 4 SERVINGS · PREP TIME: 5 minutes · COOK TIME: 5 minutes

When most people think of pudding, lemon isn't the first place their minds go, but it's a great choice. Lemon pudding is nice and light, and this version is almost like key lime pie filling. The coconut milk base offsets the tartness of the Meyer lemons while offering up a fat that the body can easily assimilate.

1 (13.66-ounce) can full-fat coconut milk

2¹/₂ tablespoons dried kudzu root, ground (see Cook's Note)

3 tablespoons Grade B maple syrup

1 tablespoon Meyer lemon zest

¹/₄ cup freshly squeezed Meyer lemon juice

¹/₄ teaspoon sea salt

1 teaspoon vanilla extract

1 pint strawberries, sliced, for garnish (optional)

Pour ¹/₂ cup the of coconut milk into a small bowl and add the kudzu. Whisk until well combined and set aside, whisking from time to time. Put the remaining coconut milk, maple syrup, lemon zest, lemon juice, salt, and vanilla into a heavy saucepan and whisk to combine. Bring to a simmer over medium heat, then whisk in the kudzu slurry. Continue to cook, whisking often, until the mixture becomes bubbly and thickened, 3 to 4 minutes. Pour into four ¹/₂-cup sized ramekins and let cool. The pudding will continue to thicken as it cools. To chill, cover with plastic pressed on the surface of the pudding. Serve with the strawberries, either warm, at room temperature, or chilled.

VARIATION: Substitute blueberries or blackberries for the strawberries.

COOK'S NOTE: Grind kudzu root with a mortar and pestle, or use a rolling pin to crush it.

PER SERVING: Serving Size: ¹/₃ cup; Calories: 131 Total Fat: 10 g (9 g saturated, 0.5 g monounsaturated); Carbohydrates: 10 g; Protein: 1 g; Fiber: 0.5 g; Sodium: 57 mg

STORAGE: Store in an airtight container in the refrigerator for up to 5 days.

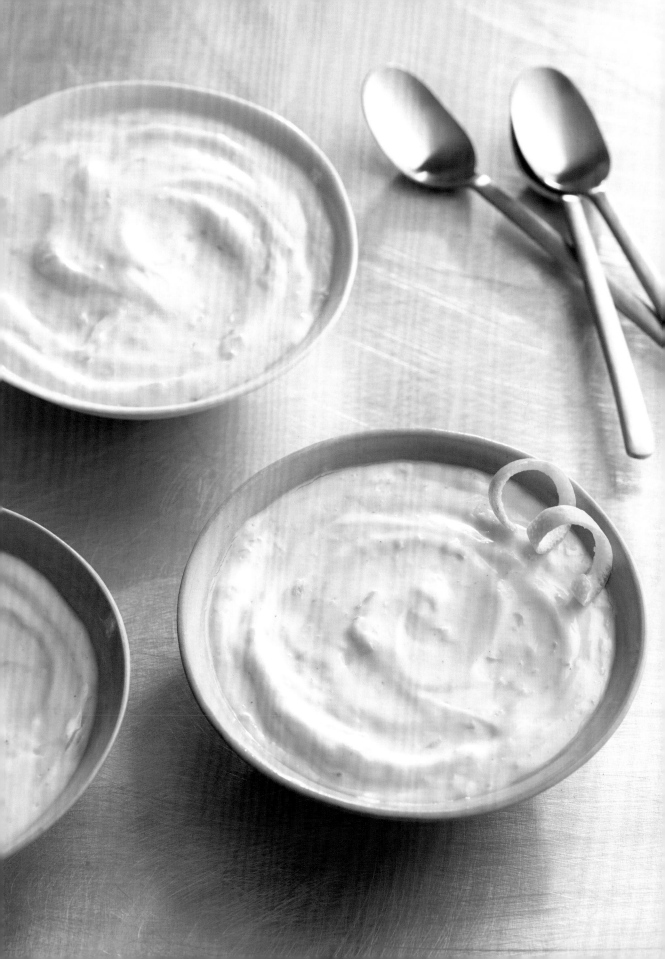

Grown-Up Chocolate Pudding
WITH RASPBERRIES

MAKES 4 SERVINGS • PREP TIME: 5 minutes • COOK TIME: 5 minutes

Talk about fun rendezvous. This little devil took a while to figure out, so my recipe tester, Catherine, and I kept meeting halfway between our homes. We'd sit in Catherine's VW bug and she'd pull out a small container of the pudding; we'd taste, figure out what needed to be tinkered with, and off we'd go on our separate ways. I wanted something that would take me back to that comforting feeling pudding gave me as a kid, yet be a little more sophisticated for an adult palate. What we ended up with was a cross between pudding, custard, and pot de crème. If that sounds a bit decadent, well, guilty as charged. Coconut milk, dark chocolate (mood enhancer!!), cinnamon, cardamom . . . yup, this one will get your motor purring.

1 (13.66-ounce) can full-fat coconut milk

1 1/2 tablespoons ground kudzu root

3 tablespoons Grade B maple syrup

1/2 teaspoon ground cinnamon

1/4 teaspoon ground cardamom

1/4 teaspoon sea salt

3 1/2 ounces dark chocolate (70% cacao), finely chopped

1 teaspoon vanilla extract

1 pint raspberries

Pour 1/2 cup of coconut milk into a small bowl and add the kudzu. Whisk until well combined and set aside, whisking from time to time. Place the remaining coconut milk, maple syrup, cinnamon, cardamom, and salt in a heavy saucepan, whisking to combine. Heat over medium flame until the mixture simmers, then whisk in the kudzu slurry. Continue to cook, whisking often, until the mixture thickens and becomes bubbly, 3 to 4 minutes. Turn off the heat and whisk in the chopped chocolate and vanilla. Pour into four 1/2-cup size ramekins. The pudding will continue to thicken as it cools. To chill, cover with plastic pressed to the surface. Serve with the raspberries either warm, room temperature, or chilled.

COOK'S NOTE: Cacao content is the amount of pure cacao in a chocolate product; the higher the percentage, the more antioxidants the chocolate contains. And if you're into addition by subtraction, higher cacao percentages also mean lower sugar content.

PER SERVING: Serving Size: 1/3 cup; Calories: 262; Total Fat: 21 g (16 g saturated, 3 g monounsaturated); Carbohydrates: 19 g; Protein: 3 g; Fiber: 2 g; Sodium: 80 mg

STORAGE: Store in an airtight container in the refrigerator for up to 5 days.

Lola's Favorite Almond Chocolate Chip Cookies

MAKES 16 COOKIES • PREP TIME: 5 minutes • COOK TIME: 15 to 17 minutes

I asked my editor if I could get away with a two-word headnote for this: "Eat these!!" But she said, "No, Rebecca. You need to say more." Sigh. How about "Eat these now!" That's what my dog Lola did. We left them on the kitchen table, wrapped in layers of parchment and foil. Lola didn't care. Her doggy delight senses shorted out her inhibition system (such as it is), and when we returned to the kitchen, she had jumped up on the table like a mountain goat and absconded with eight cookies. Fortunately, the chocolate content was low enough, and Lola big enough, that the vet said she'd be fine; she was, but there was no dinner for her that night. These are flourless, a blend of almond butter, egg, vanilla, cocoa nibs, and chocolate chips. The chocolate is guaranteed to elevate your mood. It sure elevated Lola's!

Preheat the oven to 350°F. Line a baking sheet with parchment paper or a silicone mat.

Place the almond butter, sugar, egg, vanilla, and salt in a bowl and mix well. Incorporate the chocolate chips and cocoa nibs. Using a 2-tablespoon scoop, evenly space scoops of the mixture on the baking sheet. Press down with a spatula or back of the spoon to slightly flatten. Sprinkle each cookie with a bit of fleur de sel. Bake for 15 to 17 minutes, until the cookies bounce back when touched. Cool on the baking sheet for 5 minutes, then using a spatula transfer to a cooling rack. Allow to cool for another 10 minutes.

VARIATIONS: Substitute cashew butter for the almond butter.

Substitute 1/4 cup of dried cranberries for 1/4 cup of the chocolate chips.

COOK'S NOTE: Coconut palm sugar is gaining popularity because of its naturally low glycemic load. It is produced from the nutrient-dense nectar of the tropical coconut palm tree flower, which is dried in a drum to become a delicious whole brown sugar that adds a depth of flavor and natural color. Check out the Resources (page 225) to see where this natural sweetener is available. If you don't have coconut palm sugar, you can substitute turbinado sugar.

PER SERVING: Serving Size: 1 cookie; Calories: 208; Total Fat: 12 g (3 g saturated, 6 g monounsaturated); Carbohydrates: 11 g; Protein: 4 g; Fiber: 2 g; Sodium: 32 mg

STORAGE: Store in an airtight container for up to 5 days. Freeze in an airtight container for up to 1 month.

1 cup organic unsalted almond butter

1/2 cup organic coconut palm sugar (see Cook's Note)

1 organic egg, beaten

1 teaspoon vanilla extract

1/8 teaspoon sea salt

1 cup dark chocolate chips (70% cacao)

1/4 cup cocoa nibs

1/8 teaspoon fleur de sel or another large crystal salt

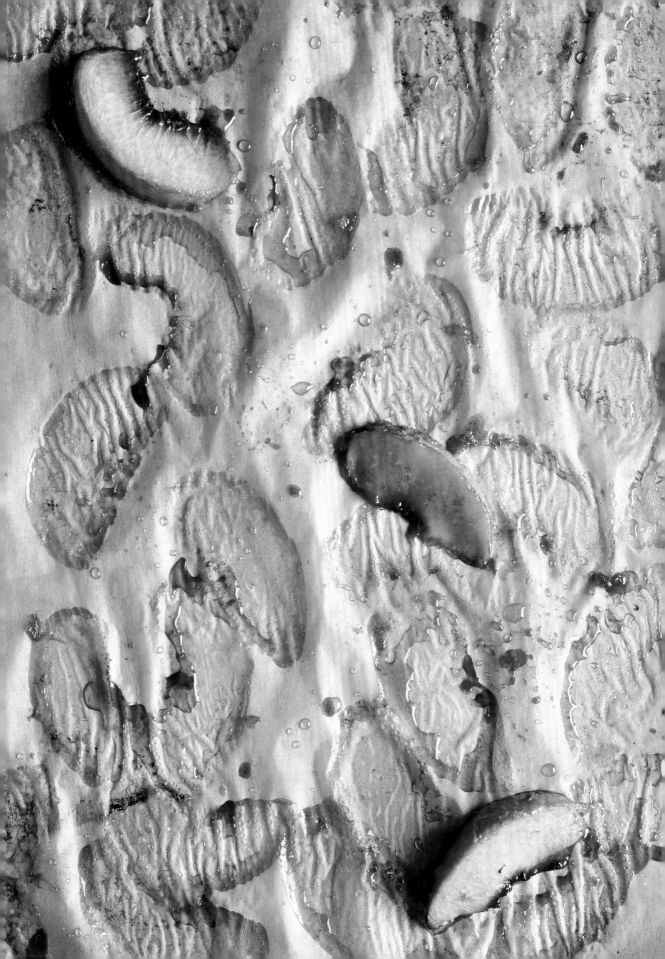

Resources

Where can you find everything from a big, sixteen-quart stockpot to heirloom rice to information on local farmers' markets? The Internet, of course. Here's a list of websites you might find useful in stocking your healthy mind pantry and staying well informed.

Specialty Ingredients

ARTISANA (for organic and raw nut butters, coconut butter, and coconut oil made in a vegan facility that processes tree nuts, but not peanuts, gluten, or soy): www.artisanafoods.com

BIG TREE FARMS (for organic coconut palm sugar; we used the blonde variety for these recipes, but vanilla would work well in the cookie recipes): www.bigtreefarms.com

BOB'S RED MILL (for teff flour, almond meal, and gluten-free oats): www.bobsredmill.com

BREAKAWAY MATCHA (for matcha green tea and frother): www.breakawaymatcha.com

CELTIC SEA SALT (for sea salt): www.selinanaturally.com

EDEN FOODS (for kombu, kudzu, dried tart cherries, and many other high-quality ingredients): www.edenfoods.com

LAKEWOOD JUICES (for organic pomegranate and blueberry juices): www.lakewoodjuices.com

LAVA LAKE LAMB (for outstanding grass-fed lamb): www.lavalakelamb.com

LIVING TREE COMMUNITY FOODS (for raw, organic, and kosher nut butters, tahini, pestos, oils, honey, and grains): www.livingtreecommunity.com

LOTUS FOODS (for heirloom and alternative varieties of rice, including forbidden rice): www.lotusfoods.com

MAINE COAST SEA VEGETABLES (for kombu): www.seaveg.com

MAPLE VALLEY (for Grade B maple syrup from an organic maple cooperative): www.maplevalleysyrup.com

MARANATHA (for organic nut and seed butters): www.maranathafoods.com

NAVITAS NATURAL (for cocoa nibs): www.navitasnaturals.com

NUMI TEA (for an organic green tea and other delicious teas): www.numitea.com

R. W. KNUDSEN (for organic juices): www.rwknudsenfamily.com

SMITH & TRUNSLOW (for freshly ground spices and spice combinations): www.smithandtruslow.com

SPECTRUM (for healthful cooking oils): www.spectrumorganics.com

TRADITIONAL MEDICINALS (for certified organic herbal and medicinal teas): www.traditionalmedicinals.com

US WELLNESS MEATS (for grass-fed and humanely raised bison, beef, chicken, and lamb): www.grasslandbeef.com

VITAL CHOICE (for wild, line-caught salmon, including lox, and other high-quality seafood; organic specialty foods; and grass-fed beef): www.vitalchoice.com

WHOLE SPICE (for "chili powder dark" blend and other amazing freshly ground herbs and spices): www.wholespice.com

National Grocery Chains and Online Markets

LOCAL HARVEST (immense directory to sources of locally grown organic food, plus an online catalog for items not available locally): www.localharvest.org

ORGANIC PROVISIONS (online organic grocery): www.orgfood.com

SAFEWAY (mainstream supermarket with its own line of organic food and produce): www.safeway.com

SPROUTS FARMERS MARKETS (chain of supermarkets in the western United States, with a focus on natural and high-quality products): www.sprouts.com

SUN ORGANIC FARM (online organic market): www.sunorganic.com

TRADER JOE'S (nationwide grocery store with organic products): www.traderjoes.com

WHOLE FOODS (the first certified organic supermarket in the United States): www.wholefoodsmarket.com

Farmers' Markets and Local Foods

EAT WELL GUIDE (directory to local, sustainable, and organic farmers' markets, restaurants, stores, bakeries, and more): www.eatwellguide.org

EAT WILD (state-by-state directory of local sources for grass-fed meats, poultry, and dairy products): www.eatwild.com

EPICURIOUS SEASONAL INGREDIENTS MAP (for info on local produce that's ripe and in season in your area at any given time): www.epicurious.com/articlesguides/seasonalcooking/farmtotable/seasonalingredientmap

LOCAL HARVEST (immense directory to sources of locally grown organic food, plus an online catalog for items not available locally): www.localharvest.org

ORGANIC KITCHEN (resource guide with listings for organic markets, restaurants, farms, vineyards, and more): www.organickitchen.com

REAL TIME FARMS (directory of local farmers and restaurants that use local foods, along with information on how food travels from field to plate): www.realtimefarms.com

US DEPARTMENT OF AGRICULTURE (nationwide farmers' market finder): http://search.ams.usda.gov/farmersmarkets/

Environmental Resources

COLLABORATIVE ON HEALTH AND THE ENVIRONMENT (for scientific research on health and the environment): www.healthandenvironment.org

ENVIRONMENTAL WORKING GROUP (for a shopper's guide to pesticides in produce): www.ewg.org/foodnews

MONTEREY BAY AQUARIUM (for a list of sustainable seafood): www.seafoodwatch.org/cr/seafoodwatch.aspx

ORGANIC CENTER (for the latest science and news about organics): www.organic-center.org

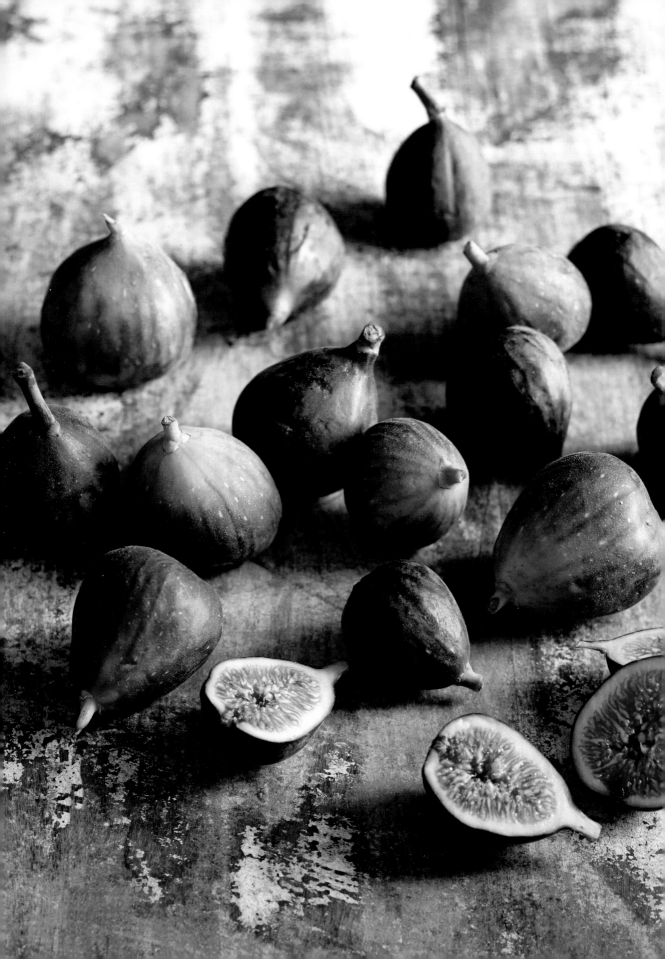

Bibliography

This bibliography represents a list of the most important, relevant, and accessible studies from the hundreds of publications consulted during the writing of this book.

Arwert, L. I., et al. 2003. Effects of an oral mixture containing glycine, glutamine and niacin on memory, GH and IGF-I secretion in middle-aged and elderly subjects. *Nutritional Neuroscience* 6(5):269–75.

Arzi, A., et al. 2004. Effect of vitamins C and E on cognitive function in mouse. *Pharmacological Research* 49(3):249–52.

Avraham, Y., et al. 2009. Capsaicin affects brain function in a model of hepatic encephalopathy associated with fulminant hepatic failure in mice. *British Journal of Pharmacology* 158(3):896–906.

Balion, C., et al. 2012. Vitamin D, cognition, and dementia: A systematic review and meta-analysis. *Neurology* 79(13):1397–1405.

Barker, S., et al. 2003. Improved performance on clerical tasks associated with administration of peppermint odor. *Perceptual and Motor Skills* 97:1007–10.

Barnard, N. 2013. *Power Foods for the Brain: A Simple, Effective Diet to Protect Your Mind and Strengthen Your Memory.* New York: Grand Central.

Belviranl, M., et al. 2013. Curcumin improves spatial memory and decreases oxidative damage in aged female rats. *Biogerontology* 14(2):187–96.

Benton, D., et al. 1997. Thiamine supplementation mood and cognitive functioning. *Psychopharmacology* 129(1):66–71.

Berr, C., et al. 2009. Olive oil and cognition: Results from the three-city study. *Dementia and Geriatric Cognitive Disorders* 28(4):357–64.

Beydoun, M. A., et al. 2007. Plasma n-3 fatty acids and the risk of cognitive decline in older adults: The Atherosclerosis Risk in Communities Study. *The American Journal of Clinical Nutrition* 85(4):1103–11.

Blondeau, N., et al. 2009. Subchronic alpha-linolenic acid treatment enhances brain plasticity and exerts an antidepressant effect: A versatile potential therapy for stroke. *Neuropsychopharmacology* 34(12):2548–59.

Borgwardt, S., et al. 2012. Neural effects of green tea extract on dorsolateral prefrontal cortex. *European Journal of Clinical Nutrition* 66(11):1187–92.

Bushara, K. O., et al. 2005. Neurologic presentation of celiac disease. *Gastroenterology* 128(4)Supplement 1: S92–7.

Carrié, I., et al. 2005. Lifelong low-phylloquinone intake is associated with cognitive impairments in old rats. *Journal of Nutrition* 141(8):1495–1501.

Castellini, C., et al. 2012. A multicriteria approach for measuring the sustainability of different poultry production systems. *Journal of Cleaner Production* 37:192–201.

Cederholm, T., et al. 2010. Are omega-3 fatty acids options for prevention and treatment of cognitive decline and dementia? *Current Opinion in Clinical Nutrition and Metabolic Care* 13(2):150–5.

Centre Hospitalier de l'Université de Montréal. 2010. Treating depression with omega-3: Encouraging results from largest clinical study. www.sciencedaily.com/releases/2010/06/100621111238.htm.

Chang, C., et al. 2009. Essential fatty acids and human brain. *Acta Neurologica Taiwanica* 18(4):231–41.

Chang, M. Y., et al. 1998/1999. Newly discovered role of retinoid receptors in high brain functions. *Journal of Medicinal Food* 1(4):299–301.

Chen, X., et al. 2012. Lower intake of vegetables and legumes associated with cognitive decline among illiterate elderly Chinese: A 3-year cohort study. *The Journal of Nutrition, Health, and Aging* 16(6):549–52.

Cherbuin, N., et al. 2014 Dietary mineral intake and risk of mild cognitive impairment: The PATH through life project. *Frontiers in Aging Neuroscience* 6:4.

Costandi, M., 2012. Does your brain produce new cells? www.theguardian.com/science/neurophilosophy/2012/feb/23/brain-new-cells-adult-neurogenesis.

Crichton, G. E., et al. 2010. Dairy intake and cognitive health in middle-aged South Australians. *Asia Pacific Journal of Clinical Nutrition* 19(2):161–71.

Dai, Q., et al. 2006. Fruit and vegetable juices and Alzheimer's disease: The Kame Project. *The American Journal of Medicine* 119(9):751–9.

Desideri, G., et al. 2012. Benefits in cognitive function, blood pressure, and insulin resistance through cocoa flavanol consumption in elderly subjects with mild cognitive impairment: The Cocoa, Cognition, and Aging (CoCoA) study. *Hypertension* 60(3):794–801.

Devore, E. E., et al. 2012. Dietary intakes of berries and flavonoids in relation to cognitive decline. *Annals of Neurology* 72(1):135–43.

Dong, S., et al. 2012. Curcumin enhances neurogenesis and cognition in aged rats: Implications for transcriptional interactions related to growth and synaptic plasticity. *PLoS ONE* 7(2).

Durga, J. et al. 2007. Effect of 3-year folic acid supplementation on cognitive function in older adults in the FACIT trial: A randomized, double blind, controlled trial. *Lancet* 369(9557):208–16.

EFSA Panel on Dietetic Products, Nutrition and Allergies (NDA). 2010. Scientific opinion on the substantiation of health claims related to riboflavin (vitamin B2) and contribution to normal energy-yielding metabolism (ID 29, 35, 36, 42), contribution to normal metabolism of iron (ID 30, 37), contribution to normal psychological functions (ID 32), maintenance of normal red blood cells (ID 40), reduction of tiredness and fatigue (ID 41), protection of DNA, proteins and lipids from oxidative damage (ID 207), and maintenance of the normal function of the nervous system (ID 213) pursuant to Article 13(1) of Regulation (EC) No 1924/2006. *EFSA Journal* 8(10): 1814–42.

Estruch, R., et al. 2013. Primary prevention of cardiovascular disease with a Mediterranean diet. *New England Journal of Medicine* 368:1279–90.

Farzaneh, A., et al. 2013. Neurovascular coupling, cerebral white matter integrity, and response to cocoa in older people. *Neurology* 81(10):904–9.

Fleenor, B. S., et al. 2013. Curcumin ameliorates arterial dysfunction and oxidative stress with aging. *Experimental Gerontology* 48(2):269–76.

Fleming, L., et al. 1994. Parkinson's disease and brain levels of organochlorine pesticides. *Annals of Neurology* 36(1):100–3.

Fragoso, Y. D., et al. 2012. High expression of retinoic acid receptors and synthetic enzymes in the human hippocampus. *Brain Structure and Function* 217(2):473–83.

Frydman-Marom, A., et al. 2011. Orally administrated cinnamon extract reduces ß-amyloid oligomerization and corrects cognitive impairment in Alzheimer's disease animal models. *PLOS One* 6(1):e16564.

Galeone, C., et al. 2009. Allium vegetable intake and risk of acute myocardial infarction in Italy. *European Journal of Nutrition* 48(2):120–23.

Gautam, S., et al. 2010. Higher bioaccessibility of iron and zinc from food grains in the presence of garlic and onion. *Journal of Agriculture and Food Chemistry* 58(14):8426–9.

Gillespie, C., et al. 2005. Hypercortisolemia and depression. *Psychosomatic Medicine* 67(Supplement 1):S26–S28.

Gordon, J. 2008. *Unstuck: Your Guide to the Seven-Stage Journey Out of Depression.* New York: Penguin.

Gorinstein, S., et al. 2006. Red grapefruit positively influences serum triglyceride level in patients suffering from coronary atherosclerosis: Studies in vitro and in humans. *Journal of Agricultural and Food Chemistry* 54(5):1887–92.

Graham, T., et al. 2011. *The Happiness Diet: A Nutritional Prescription for a Sharp Brain, Balanced Mood, and Lean, Energized Body.* New York: Rodale.

Greger, M. 2012. How to Boost Serotonin Naturally. http://nutritionfacts.org/2012/11/15/boost-serotonin-naturally/.

Haider, S., et al. 2008. Repeated administration of fresh garlic increases memory retention in rats. *Journal of Medicinal Food* 11(4):675–9.

Harada, N., et al. 2009. Stimulation of sensory neurons improves cognitive function by promoting the hippocampal production of insulin-like growth factor-I in mice. *Translational Research* 154(2):90–102.

Harrison, F. E. 2012. A critical review of vitamin C for the prevention of age-related cognitive decline and Alzheimer's disease. *Journal of Alzheimer's Disease* 29(4):711–26.

Held, K., et al. 2002. Oral Mg^{2+} supplementation reverses age-related neuroendocrine and sleep eeg changes in humans. *Pharmacopsychiatry* 35(4):135–43.

Heo, H., et al. 2006. Phenolic phytochemicals in cabbage inhibit amyloid ß protein-induced neurotoxicity. *LWT–Food Science and Technology* 39(4):331–37.

Holland, E. 2011. Omega-3 reduces anxiety and inflammation in healthy students. http://researchnews.osu.edu/archive/omega3.htm.

Howatson, G., et al. 2012. Effect of tart cherry juice (*Prunus cerasus*) on melatonin levels and enhanced sleep quality. *European Journal of Nutrition* 51(8):909–16.

Hwang, I. K., et al. 2009. Neuroprotective effects of onion extract and quercetin against ischemic neuronal damage in the gerbil hippocampus. *Journal of Medicinal Food* 12(5):990–95.

Hyman, M. 2008. *The UltraMind Solution: Fix Your Broken Brain by Healing Your Body First.* New York: Scribner.

Jana, A., et al. 2013. Up-regulation of neurotrophic factors by cinnamon and its metabolite sodium benzoate: Therapeutic implications for neurodegenerative disorders. *Journal of Neuroimmune Pharmacology* 8(3):739–55.

Jang, S., et al. 2010. Luteolin inhibits microglia and alters hippocampal-dependent spatial working memory in aged mice. *Journal of Nutrition* 140(10):1892–8.

Jensen, K. M., et al. 2004. Intakes of whole grains, bran, and germ and the risk of coronary heart disease in men. *American Journal of Clinical Nutrition* 80(6):1492–99.

Jittiwat, J., et al. 2012. Ginger pharmacopuncture improves cognitive impairment and oxidative stress following cerebral ischemia. *Journal of Acupuncture and Meridian Studies* 5(6):295–300.

Joosten, H., et al. 2013. Cardiovascular risk profile and cognitive function in young, middle-aged, and elderly subjects. *Stroke* 44(6):1543–9.

Kalmijn, S., et al. 2004. Dietary intake of fatty acids and fish in relation to cognitive performance at middle age. *Neurology* 62(2):275–80.

Kanarek, R. B., et al. 1990. Effects of food snacks on cognitive performance in male college students. *Appetite* 14(1): 15-27.

Kelly, J. H. Jr., et al. 2006. Nuts and coronary heart disease: An epidemiological perspective. *British Journal of Nutrition* 96 Supplement 2:S61–7.

Khan, M., et al. 2006. Prevention of cognitive impairments and neurodegeneration by Khamira Abresham Hakim Arshad Wala. *Journal of Ethnopharmacology* 108(1):68–73.

Kim, J. M., et al. 2008. Changes in folate, vitamin B12 and homocysteine associated with incident dementia. *Journal of Neurology, Neurosurgery, and Psychiatry* 79(8):864–8.

Koppula, S., et al. 2011. Cuminum cyminum extract attenuates scopolamine-induced memory loss and stress-induced urinary biochemical changes in rats: A noninvasive biochemical approach. *Pharmaceutical Biology* 49(7):702–8.

Kuriyama, S., et al. 2006. Green tea consumption and cognitive function: A cross-sectional study from the Tsurugaya Project 123. *American Journal of Clinical Nutrition* 83(2):355–61.

Landfield, P., et al. 1984. Chronically elevating plasma Mg^{2+} improves hippocampal frequency potentiation and reversal learning in aged and young rats. *Brain Research* 322(1):167–71.

Landgraph, T., et al. 2013. Nutrient composition of poultry from different farms and management systems. *Practical Farmers of Iowa,* January 2013: (1-4)

Letenneur, L., et al. 2007. Flavonoid intake and cognitive decline over a 10-year period. *American Journal of Epidemiology* 165(12):1364–71.

Lindeman, R., et al. 2000. Serum vitamin B12, C and folate concentrations in the New Mexico Elder Health Survey: correlations with cognitive and affective functions. *Journal of the American College of Nutrition* 19(1):68–76.

Llewellyn, D. J., et al. 2010. Vitamin D and risk of cognitive decline in elderly persons. *JAMA Internal Medicine (formerly Archives of Internal Medicine)*: 170(13):1135-41.

Low, J. W., et al. 2007. A food-based approach introducing orange-fleshed sweet potatoes increased vitamin A intake and serum retinol concentrations in young children in rural Mozambique. *Journal of Nutrition* 137(5):1320–7.

Lu, J., et al. 2012. Purple sweet potato color attenuates domoic acid-induced cognitive deficits by promoting estrogen receptor-ß-mediated mitochondrial biogenesis signaling in mice. *Free Radical Biology and Medicine* 52(3):646–59.

Lupien, S. J., et al. 2007. The effects of stress and stress hormones on human cognition: Implications for the field of brain and cognition. *Brain and Cognition* 65:231: 434–445.

Macready, A. L., et al. 2009 Flavonoids and cognitive function: A review of human randomized controlled trial studies and recommendations for future studies. *Genes & Nutrition* 4(4):227–42.

Mahoney, C. R., et al. 2005. Effect of breakfast composition on cognitive processes in elementary school children. *Physiology & Behavior* 85(5):635–45.

Mangialasche, F., et al. 2012. Tocopherols and tocotrienols plasma levels are associated with cognitive impairment. *Neurobiology of Aging* 33(10):2282–90.

Mani, V., et al. 2011. Reversal of memory deficits by *Coriandrum sativum* leaves in mice. *Journal of the Science of Food and Agriculture* 91(1):186–92.

Matchynski, J., et al. 2013. Combinatorial treatment of tart cherry extract and essential fatty acids reduces cognitive impairments and inflammation in the mu-p75 saporin-induced mouse model of Alzheimer's disease. *Journal of Medicinal Food* 16(4):288–95.

McGrath, M. 2013. EU says pesticides may harm human brains. www.bbc.com/news/science-environment-25421199.

Mechan, A., et al. 2010. Monoamine reuptake inhibition and mood-enhancing potential of a specified oregano extract. *British Journal of Nutrition* 105(8):1150–63.

Milind, P., et al. 2012. Anti-Alzheimer's potential of orange juice. *International Research Journal of Pharmacy* 3(9):312–16.

Mohajeri, M. H., et al. 2012. Modulation of neurotransmission by a specified oregano extract alters brain electrical potentials indicative of antidepressant-like and neuroprotective activities. *Neuroscience & Medicine* 3(1):37–46.

Moorthy, D., et al. 2012. Status of vitamins B12 and B6 but not of folate, homocysteine, and the methylenetetrahydrofolate reductase C677T polymorphism are associated with impaired cognition and depression in adults. *Journal of Nutrition* 142(8):1554–60.

Morgan, J. M., et al. 2002. Effects of walnut consumption as part of a low-fat, low-cholesterol diet on serum cardiovascular risk factors. *International Journal for Vitamin and Nutritional Research* 72(5):341–47.

Morris, M. C., et al. 2004. Dietary niacin and the risk of incident Alzheimer's disease and of cognitive decline. *Journal of Neurology, Neurosurgery, and Psychiatry* 75:1093–99.

Moss, M., et al. 2008. Modulation of cognitive performance and mood by aromas of peppermint and ylang-ylang. *International Journal of Neuroscience* 118(1):59–77.

Mullen, W., et al. 2007. Evaluation of phenolic compounds in commercial fruit juices and fruit drinks. *Journal of Agricultural and Food Chemistry* 55(8):3148–57.

Mullin, G., et al. 2011. *The Inside Tract: Your Good Gut Guide to Great Digestive Heath.* New York: Rodale.

Murray-Kolb, L. E., et al. 2007. Iron treatment normalizes cognitive functioning in young women. *American Journal of Clinical Nutrition* 85(3):778–87.

Nooyens, A. C., et al. 2011. Fruit and vegetable intake and cognitive decline in middle-aged men and women: The Doetinchem Cohort Study. *British Journal of Nutrition* 106(5):752–61.

Okereke, O., et al. 2012. Dietary fat types and 4-year cognitive change in community-dwelling older women. *Annals of Neurology* 72(1):124–34.

Olson, C. R., et al. 2010. Significance of vitamin A to brain function, behavior, and learning. *Molecular Nutrition and Food Research* 54(4):489–95.

Oude, Griep, L. M. et al., 2011. Colours of fruit and vegetables and 10-year incidence of CHD. *British Journal of Nutrition* 106(10):1562–9.

Page, K., et al. 2008. *The Flavor Bible: The Essential Guide to Culinary Creativity, Based on the Wisdom of America's Most Imagiative Chefs.* New York: Little, Brown.

Pan, E., et al. 2011. Vesicular zinc promotes presynaptic and inhibits postsynaptic long-term potentiation of mossy fiber-CA3 synapse. *Neuron* 71(6):1116–26.

Park, S. K., et al. 2011. A combination of green tea extract and l-theanine improves memory and attention in subjects with mild cognitive impairment: A double-blind placebo-controlled study. *Journal of Medicinal Food* 14(4):334–43.

Perry, S. 2011. A matter of taste. www .brainfacts.org/Sensing-Thinking-Behaving/ Senses-and-Perception/Articles/2011/ A-Matter-of-Taste

Perlmutter, D., et al. 2013. *Grain Brain: The Surprising Truth about Wheat, Carbs, and Sugar—Your Brain's Silent Killers.* New York: Little, Brown.

Pigeon, W. R., et al. 2010. Effects of a tart cherry juice beverage on the sleep of older adults with insomnia: A pilot study. *Journal of Medicinal Food* 13(3):579–83.

Poly, C., et al. 2011. The relation of dietary choline to cognitive performance and white-matter hyperintensity in the Framingham Offspring Cohort. *American Journal of Clinical Nutrition* 94(6):1584–91.

Presse, N., et. al. 2013. Vitamin K status and cognitive function in healthy older adults. *Neurobiology of Aging* 34(12):2777–83.

Rasgon, N. L., et al. 2005. Insulin resistance in depressive disorders and Alzheimer's disease: Revisiting the missing link hypothesis. *Neurobiology of Aging* 26, Supplement 1:103–7.

Rahman, K., et al. 2003. Garlic and aging: new insights into an old remedy. *Aging Research Reviews* 2(1):39–56.

Reger, M. A., et al. 2004. Effects of beta-hydroxybutyrate on cognition in memory-impaired adults. *Neurobiology of Aging* 25(3):311–4.

Reiter, R. J., et al. 2005. Melatonin in walnuts: Influence on levels of melatonin and total antioxidant capacity of blood. *Nutrition* 21(9):920–4.

Robinson, J. G., et al. 2010. Omega-3 fatty acids and cognitive function in women. *Women's Health* 6(1):119–34.

Ros, E. 2010. Health benefits of nut consumption. *Nutrients* 2(7):652–82.

Saenghong, N., et al. 2011. Ginger supplementation enhances working memory of the post-menopause woman. *American Journal of Applied Science* 8(12):1241–48.

Saenghong, N., et al. 2012. *Zingiber officinale* improves cognitive function of the middle-aged healthy women. *Evidence-Based Complementary and Alternative Medicine.* http://www.hindawi.com/journals/ecam/2012/383062/

Sakakibara, H., et al. 2008. Antidepressant-like effect of onion (*Allium cepa L.*) powder in a rat behavioral model of depression. *Bioscience, Biotechnology & Biochemistry* 72(1):94–100.

Sarter, M., et al. 2005. Choline transporters, cholinergic transmission, and cognition. *Nature Reviews Neuroscience* 6(1):48–56.

Schafer, J. H., et al. 2005. Homocysteine and cognitive function in a population-based study of older adults. *Journal of American Geriatric Society* 53(3):381–8.

Scott, K. 2006. *Medicinal Seasonings: The Healing Power of Spices.* Cape Town, South Africa: Medspice.

Serafini, M., et al. 2003. Plasma antioxidants from chocolate. *Nature* 424(6952):1013.

Silaste, M. L., et al. 2007. Tomato juice decreases LDL cholesterol levels and increases LDL resistance to oxidation. *British Journal of Nutrition* 98(6):1251–8.

Simopoulos, A., et al. 1999. *The Omega Diet: The Lifesaving Nutritional Program Based on the Diet of the Island of Crete.* New York: Harper.

Slutsky, I., et al. 2010. Enhancement of learning and memory by elevating brain magnesium. *Neuron* 65(2):165–77.

Spencer, J. P. 2008. Food for thought: The role of dietary flavonoids in enhancing human memory, learning, and neurocognitive performance. *Proceedings of the Nutrition Society* 67(2):238–52.

Stromberg, J. 2014. A scientific explanation of how marijuana causes the munchies. www.smithsonianmag.com/science-nature/scientific-explanation-how-marijuana-causes-munchies-180949660/.

Swardfager, W., et al. 2013. Zinc in depression: A meta-analysis. *Biological Psychiatry* 74(12):872–78.

Tangney, C. C., et al. 2009. Biochemical indicators of vitamin B12 and folate insufficiency and cognitive decline. *Neurology* 72(4):361–367.

Taste and smell. 2012. http://www.brain facts.org/Sensing-Thinking-Behaving/Senses-and-Perception/Articles/2012/Taste-and-Smell.

Tian, M., et al. 2012. Curcumin preserves cognitive function and improve serum HDL in chronic cerebral hypoperfusion aging-rats. *Molecular Neurodegeneration* 7, Supplement 1:S3.

Tildesley, N. T., et al. 2014. *Salvia lavandulaefolia* (Spanish sage) enhances memory in healthy young volunteers. *Pharmacology, Biochemistry & Behavior* 75(3):669–74.

Tribole, E. 2007. *The Ultimate Omega-3 Diet: Maximize the Power of Omega-3s to Supercharge Your Health, Battle Inflammation, and Keep Your Mind Sharp.* New York: McGraw Hill.

Trivedi, B. 2012. Neuroscience: Hardwired for taste. *Nature,* June 12:S7–S9.

Tucker, K. L., et al. 2005. High homocysteine and low B vitamins predict cognitive decline in aging men: The Veterans Affairs Normative Aging Study. *American Journal of Clinical Nutrition* 82(3):627–25.

Tulane University. 2013. High blood sugar makes Alzheimer's plaque more toxic to the brain. *ScienceDaily*, October 29.

Valls-Pedret, C., et al. 2012. Polyphenol-rich foods in the Mediterranean diet are associated with better cognitive function in elderly subjects at high cardiovascular risk. *Journal of Alzheimer's Disease* 29(4):773–82.

Vauzour, D., et al. 2008. The neuroprotective potential of flavonoids: A multiplicity of effects. *Genes & Nutrition* 3(3–4):115–26.

Vinot, N., et al. 2011. Omega-3 fatty acids from fish oil lower anxiety, improve cognitive functions and reduce spontaneous locomotor activity in a non-human primate. *PLoS ONE* 6(6).

Walker, J. G., et al. 2011. Oral folic acid and vitamin B12 supplementation to prevent cognitive decline in community-dwelling older adults with depressive symptoms— the Beyond Aging Project: A randomized controlled trial. *The American Journal of Clinical Nutrition.*

Wang, Y., et al. 2012. Green tea epigallocatechin-3-gallate (EGCG) promotes neural progenitor cell proliferation and sonic hedgehog pathway activation during adult hippocampal neurogenesis. *Molecular Nutrition and Food Research* 56(8):1292–1303.

Wärnberg, J. 2009. Nutrition, inflammation, and cognitive function. *Annals of the New York Academy of Science* 1153:164–75.

Weil, A. 2011 *Depression and the Anti-Inflammatory Diet.* Video. http://drweil.com/drw/u/VDR00040/Depression-and-the-Anti-Inflammatory-Diet.html.

Weil, A. 2011. *Spontaneous Happiness.* New York: Little, Brown.

Wenk, G. 2012. Can the Mediterranean diet treat your depression? www.psychology today.com/blog/your-brain-food/201205/can-the-mediterranean-diet-treat-your-depression.

Wenk, G. 2010. *Your Brain on Food: How Chemicals Control Your Thoughts and Feelings.* New York: Oxford University Press.

Willis, L. M., et al. 2009. Dose-dependent effects of walnuts on motor and cognitive function in aged rats. *British Journal of Nutrition* 101(8):1140–4.

Wilson, A. 2012. Slash chronic disease risk with lycopene. *Life Extension Magazine, December.*

Wu, A., et al. 2004. Dietary omega-3 fatty acids normalize BDNF levels, reduce oxidative damage, and counteract learning disability after traumatic brain injury in rats. *Journal of Neurotrauma* 21(10):1457–67.

Wu, D. M., et al. 2013. Ursolic acid improves domoic acid-induced cognitive deficits in mice. *Toxicology and Applied Pharmacology* 271(2):127–36.

Wurtman, J. 2009. *The Serotonin Power Diet: Eat Carbs—Natures Own Appetite Suppressant—to Stop Emotional Overeating and Halt Antidepressant-Associated Weight Gain.* New York, Rodale.

Youdim, M. B. 2008. Brain iron deficiency and excess: Cognitive impairment and neurodegeneration with involvement of striatum and hippocampus. *Neurotoxicity Research* 14(1):45–56.

Young, S. N., et al. 2007. How to increase serotonin in the human brain without drugs. *Journal of Psychiatry and Neuroscience* 32(6):394–9.

Zhang, M., et al. 2011. Vitamin C provision improves mood in acutely hospitalized patients. *Nutrition* 27(5):530–3.

Zoladz, P., et al. 2005. Cognitive enhancement through stimulation of the chemical senses. *North American Journal of Psychology* 7(1):125–40.

Zomer, E., et al. 2012. The effectiveness and cost effectiveness of dark chocolate consumption as prevention therapy in people at high risk of cardiovascular disease: Best case scenario analysis using a Markov model. *British Medical Journal*; 344:e3657.

Zotti, M., et al. 2013. Carvacrol: From ancient flavoring to neuromodulatory agent. *Molecules* 18(6):6161–72.

Index

For my remarkable mother, Barbara P. Katz
In memory of my much-loved father, Joseph J. Katz

Published in the United States by Ten Speed Press, an imprint of
the Crown Publishing Group, a division of Random House LLC,
a Penguin Random House Company, New York.
www.crownpublishing.com
www.tenspeed.com

Ten Speed Press and the Ten Speed Press colophon are registered
trademarks of Random House LLC.

Library of Congress Cataloging-in-Publication Data
Katz, Rebecca.
  The healthy mind cookbook : big-flavor recipes to enhance brain function,
mood, memory, and mental clarity / Rebecca Katz, Mat Edelson ; photography
by Maren Caruso.
     pages cm
1. Brain. 2. Mental health—Nutritional aspects. 3. Intellect—Nutritional aspects.
4. Cooking. I. Edelson, Mat. II. Caruso, Maren. III. Title.
  QP376.K344 2015
  641.5'63--dc23

                              2014025924

Hardcover ISBN: 978-1-60774-297-5
eBook ISBN: 978-1-60774-298-2

Printed in China

Design by Chloe Rawlins
Food styling by Christine Wolheim
Prop styling by Kerrie Sherrel Walsh

10 9 8 7 6 5 4

First Edition